Dr. Moyad's

GUIDE TO

Male Sexual Health

What Works And What's Worthless

Mark A. Moyad, MD, MPH

This edition is published by Spry Publishing LLC

2500 South State Street

Ann Arbor, MI 48104 USA

www.sprypub.com

Printed and bound in the US.

Library of Congress Cataloging-in-Publication Data on file.

ISBN: 978-1-938170-01-0

10   9   8   7   6   5   4   3   2   1

Contents

Introduction

For the past fifteen years, I have maintained a consulting practice in complementary medicine. I've become known as an expert in over-the-counter natural medicines and have helped both individuals and healthcare professionals sort through choices to determine what works and what is worthless. I speak internationally on the topic of complementary medicine and particularly on issues related to men's sexual health and prostate cancer. This book is a direct result of the many, many conversations that I have had with men and their partners on my travels.

You see, it became painfully clear to me in talking with men that there is a real need for some frank conversation on the topic of male sexual health. Men are often uncomfortable and hesitant to speak about such a personal issue with their partners, their friends, and often, sadly, even with their health care providers.

This book is an effort to take a candid look at the topic in a lighthearted fashion in order to convince men that, like life, sexual health education should be enjoyable and that there are plenty of costly and not-so-costly options available. As you read the book, I hope that you will take away a number of simple lifestyle changes that can really improve your sexual health. If you have questions or need additional help, please seek the advice of your primary care provider, or possibly a specialist, such as a urologist, endocrinologist, gynecologist, psychologist, nutritionist, or social worker. Although it may be a difficult conversation to begin, the dialog gets easier once started, and think of the possible rewards! There is no doubt that your sexual health impacts your overall well being and health, too. Now is the time to begin your journey toward an improved sex life—read on!

Mark A. Moyad, MD, MPH

CHAPTER 1

Dr. Moyad's Favorite Myths, Misconceptions, and Facts About Sexual Enhancement

I thought we'd start off by playing a game of true-or-false to test what you know about sexual health. As with magazine survey questions, you get to keep your own score and you can tally as honestly (or dishonestly!) as you choose. However, you'll find hundreds of fun facts tucked into our little game. See how you score!

QUESTION 1
Is it true that the penis is the best barometer of a man's overall health?

TRUE!
I constantly chuckle at experts and self-help books that try and convince the public that there is some magical sexual health diet. Wrong! The same diet and routine that promotes heart health actually is the best diet to make the penis work the best and to enhance your sexual life. Think about all the things that are bad for the heart and then consider the ones that can damage the penis and your sex life (male or female):

Alcohol (more than moderate consumption)
Anxiety and emotional upset (guilt, low self-esteem, fear, etc.)
Bad diet
Blood disorders (anemia)
Cardiovascular disease
Depression
Hormonal abnormalities (prolactin, testosterone, thyroid, etc.)
High blood glucose (diabetes)
High blood pressure (hypertension)
High cholesterol (higher LDL and/or triglycerides)
Kidney disease
Lack of exercise
Lack of sleep and obstructive sleep apnea
Low amount of "good" cholesterol (low HDL)
Medication use (some prescriptions and over-the-counter medicines)
Neurologic diseases

Penile abnormalities (Peyronie's disease)

Peripheral vascular disease (PAD)

Prostate problems (cancer treatment, enlargement, infection, inflammation, etc.)

Smoking (or smokeless tobacco use)

Substance abuse (marijuana use included)

Stress

Trauma or surgery to the pelvis or spine

Weight or waist gain

See how many of the heart "risks" are also on the sexual health risk list?

Also, erectile or sexual dysfunction can be an indicator of a future life-threatening disease, especially in younger men. The types of cells that line the heart or blood vessels are similar to the ones that line the penis. The blood vessels that supply the penis (penile artery) are 1 to 2 millimeters in diameter, the blood vessels that supply the heart (coronary artery) are 3 to 5 millimeters in diameter, and the blood vessels that supply the brain (carotid artery) are 4 to 6 millimeters in diameter. Many researchers suggests that the penis runs into trouble before the heart does because the vessels that lead to the penis are smaller and more vulnerable to damage. If a man has erectile issues early in life, many doctors will refer him to a cardiologist, and I could not agree more with this course of action. Cardiovascular disease is both the number-one killer of men and women and the number-one cause of sexual dysfunction in men! Paying special attention to your penis may just be important for your heart, too!

QUESTION 2
Is it true that an erection involves the concerted and coordinated actions of the brain and spinal cord (nervous system), blood vessels, and hormones?

TRUE! TRUE! TRUE!
This is why even a small abnormal function in one of these coordinated areas can cause problems, and also why sexual problems are so common. Let's review the actual effort involved in creating an erection (sound like a trip back to health education class?). The non-erect (flaccid) penis is under venous (as in vein) oxygen tension and pressure, which means not much is going on at the amusement park because the doors are not open yet. Erotic stimulation occurs, triggered by any one of many things. The brain and nervous system respond by quickly sending messages to the pelvic area causing the smooth muscles in the penis to relax. The blood vessels in the penis open wider due to compounds that are released, such as nitric oxide (NO), and this increases the blood flow into two parallel sponge-like cylinders (the corpora cavernosa), which run along the length of the penis on both sides. The corpora cavernosa are above the urethra, the passageway for urine and semen. As the cylinders fill with blood, they expand and press against the veins that would usually drain blood from the penis. This causes the penis

to lengthen and swell, resulting in an erection (also called "tumescence"). During an erection, the penis is an arterial organ because fresh oxygenated blood has been pumped into it. After ejaculation or when sexual arousal has passed, the nervous system releases norepinephrine and other compounds, and blood actually drains out of the cylinders in the penis. The penis returns to its original size and shape (also called "detumescence"). And, you thought an erection was such a simple task! It takes a lot to keep that amusement park open for business (except for 18-year-olds, whose amusement parks ALWAYS seem to be up and running!).

QUESTION 3
Are strong morning erections, spontaneous erections, and more interest in sex in the morning a healthy sign?

TRUE! TRUE! TRUE!
Men who get erections in the morning should be congratulated. Men tend to experience their highest daily blood levels of testosterone or a surge in testosterone in the early to mid-morning (generally around 6 to 8 AM). Testosterone is one of the primary hormones that helps put men in the mood and helps to make the male equipment stand tall. Morning erections and an increased sex drive are good indicators that the machinery and the circuits to the machinery are working well! Health-care professionals are well aware of the testosterone peak and generally test blood testosterone levels no later than 9 AM. Determining the maximum hormone release is an important piece of information in assessing a man's sexual health.

Generally speaking, there is a reduction in blood levels of total testosterone at a rate of about one percent per year after the age of 30 years. In fact, some researchers have used the term "andropause" ("andro" meaning male) to describe the slow loss of testosterone over decades. Unlike female menopause, which results from the rapid loss of estrogen over several years, andropause is a gradual process. Also dissimilarly, when men lose weight their testosterone levels generally increase, and when women lose weight their levels of estrogen slightly decrease. Seems odd, but it is true!

Morning erections are so common that doctors use the presence or absence of a nocturnal erection as a sign of your potential sexual health. If you don't experience them regularly, then discuss this fact with your doctor at your next visit. If they are a regular occurrence for you, then celebrate in some appropriate fashion of your choosing!

QUESTION 4
What is "average" for penis size?

The average penis size (not stretched) ranges from 3.5 (8.85 cm) to 4.2 inches (10.7 cm), and the average stretched penis size ranges from 4.9 (12.45 cm) to 6.6 inches (16.74 cm). The average erection length ranges from 5.1 (12.89 cm)

⌐ inches (15.5 cm). It turns out that there is no good predictor of erect penis ᵴ. —not hand size, not foot size, not the size of the non-erect penis—except for perhaps height and seeing someone naked with an erection.

These dimensions come from results of most of the previous studies on penis size, where ages ranged from 17 to 91 years old! I know what you are thinking ... you need to run out immediately and buy yourself a tape measure because you have some important work around the house that needs to get done! By the way, there have also been average penis (mid-shaft) circumference studies of the non-erect and erect penis, which is between 3.8 (9.71 cm) and 4.8 inches.

Keep in mind that every person has a pubic fat pad, which tends to increase with age and weight/waist gain. It can draw the penis in toward the abdomen and essentially "shrink" the penis. So, are we saying that penile length decreases with age? The answer is that it depends on whether or not your belly fat is increasing with age. If you want to keep your penis a similar size to when you were young buck, please try and prevent belly fat or your waist size from increasing. I know this is not easy, but it keeps me jumping on the treadmill at least 5 to 7 days a week.

QUESTION 5
Can a man can have an orgasm without an erection?

TRUE!
Seems strange, doesn't it? We obviously know that men can have an erection without an orgasm. However, an orgasm without an erection again demonstrates the complexity of the male erection and male sexuality. For example, some men who suffer from damage to the nerves that control erections are able to have an orgasm without an erection when adequately stimulated. Other men have the equivalent of a "wet dream" without an erection while they are awake and mentally stimulated. Granted, this is a minority of adult men, but it is interesting to note our similarities and differences when it comes to sexual health.

QUESTION 6
Is there something I can do to up the odds of having intense orgasms?

TRUE!
Women and men can actually increase the strength of their pelvic floor muscles with Kegel exercises that are easy to do. First, start by tightly squeezing and fully releasing your pubococcygeus muscle 10 times (say that 4 times fast while eating saltines). The easiest possible way to find and isolate this muscle is to simply to try and stop your flow of urine (without using your hands please) the next time you go to the bathroom. Once you've located the muscle, do several sets of the tightening exercise, with a 10- to 20-second break in between. Repeat 2 to 3 times

a day. As your pelvic muscles become stronger, try to hold that tight squeeze for longer. You can do this anywhere—watching television, waiting in line, or driving in your car. You will actually feel the results of your minimal (surreptitious to the public) workout within several weeks. It may help women have multiple or more intense orgasms and could also help men have more intense orgasms.

Any other exercises that increase flexibility and strengthen the stabilizing muscles in your lower body, pelvis, and core can enhance your sex life and certainly can help you twist and turn in varied sexual positions. Flexibility and core strength are not only heart healthy but important for sexual health.

QUESTION 7
Is it true that more ejaculations and orgasms can also prevent certain diseases?

PROBABLY TRUE! (Perhaps worth lying about if it were not true!)
In one of the largest studies in the world ever completed considering ejaculations and prostate cancer, men who had the highest average number of ejaculations (ejaculation frequency) per month experienced the largest reduction in the risk of prostate cancer. In fact, men who reported that they had 21 or more ejaculations per month actually had the largest reductions in the occurrence of prostate cancer. (21 per month! Perhaps lying reduces the risk of prostate cancer?) Look, 21 or more ejaculations would just make me sleepy and dehydrated!

And, speaking of being sleepy, men release more sleep-inducing hormones (oxytocin, prolactin, etc.) after an orgasm. It appears that there is a physiological reason why we are not so good at cuddling, but experts at snoozing, after a sexual experience.

Other studies suggest a variety of health benefits from regular ejaculations. Is this due to the flushing of carcinogens that come into contact with the prostate (similar to the way consumption of fluids might reduce the risk of bladder cancer)? A positive note for those men who want to have more ejaculations to reduce their risk of prostate cancer (and their partners, actually): self-induced and nocturnal ejaculations (wet dreams) are usually counted in the monthly ejaculation total. Any means to better health, I suppose!

QUESTION 8
Can just a few pounds of weight loss equal more testosterone, sex drive, and erections?

TRUE!
Just a few pounds of weight loss or removing a few inches from your waist can increase a man's testosterone immediately and increase his sex drive and erectile

function. Yes, by the way, it has a tendency to do the same thing for some women.

Experts who love to push expensive prescription options and over-the-counter (OTC) pills, pills, pills, and more pills as a solution for sexual dysfunction or sex drive tend to discount the benefits that can be achieved by simply losing weight. This technique is cheap, has no negative side effects (unless you count that losing weight is always going to be a pain in the ass itself), and should always be a part of any sexual enhancement program.

QUESTION 9
Is the skin the most underappreciated sexual organ?

TRUE!
It is the largest organ of the body (not the penis, you egomaniacs). It has a surface area of about 15 feet and has sensitive nerve endings or receptors that respond to all kinds of feelings and emotions. Sensual touch, kissing, and sucking can contribute to arousal or lubrication without even touching the genitals. And, skin-to-skin contact stimulates the production of the hormone oxytocin and releases endorphins, which increases bonding and pleasure. The nose, eyelids, and lips are among the most sensitive spots on the body, as are the ears (outside and inside), the inner thighs, the small of the back, and the area under the belly button. Those areas have a thin layer of skin with a lot of receptors underneath them. Other neglected zones of stimulation include the sides of the neck, the underside of the wrists, the perineum (area between the vagina and anus), the anus itself, the toes, and between the toes. Many of these areas of the skin transmit messages to the brain's sexual centers that then transmit a message to the genitals to prepare for sexual activity.

Interestingly, women are 5 to 10 times more sensitive to touch as compared to men, which means men or other women need to consider this fact more when trying to arouse a female partner. Some of you (hopefully a small number) are unfortunately thinking that some of these areas are gross to touch with your hand or mouth. You could not be more wrong! You should be more concerned about getting a yearly flu shot because the flu kills 36,000 people and hospitalizes 200,000 every year in the United States alone. I have yet to hear of anyone who died from nibbling on his partner's toes.

QUESTION 10
Which one of the following is true?

Sex makes you look younger.
Sex burns calories.
Sex reduces pain.
Sex helps you breathe easier.

Sex can help your body fight diseases.
Sex promotes a feeling of overall relationship and personal well being.
Sex helps you live longer.

ALL ARE TRUE!

Recent research shows that sex reduces stress and gives you better sleep, both of which make you feel more youthful. It burns about 100 to 150 calories in 20 minutes, which means the beer or wine you drank at dinner was not a caloric problem. Natural painkillers are released during sex (similar to a "runner's high"), and there are increases in natural antihistamines and immunoglobulin A, which allow you to breathe easier and keep your immune system functioning well. Sex causes surges in natural calming compounds of the body and relationship-bonding hormones such as oxytocin and endorphins, especially when an orgasm occurs, which is why it is easy to fall asleep happy after sexual activity. And, regular sex increases the chance that other areas of your health will get more attention (sleep, stress, cholesterol, exercise), which means an increased chance to live longer!

QUESTION 11
Are men really visual animals?

TRUE!

Why do men asked to provide a sperm sample in a cup get "dirty" magazines or films? Let's finally just admit that men are incredibly visual animals!

That means that a partner who likes to dress up and look good may be more sexually attractive. It may also mean that sharing some suggestive images or an off-color film isn't a bad idea if both partners enjoy the activity.

Here's your secret tip of the day—men aren't the only visual creatures in the bedroom. Some women may be hesitant to admit it, but research shows that they can be every bit as aroused by a well-rounded body!

QUESTION 12
Can women have multiple orgasms? How about men?

TRUE and NOT REALLY!

Women have some advantages over men besides their ability to ask for directions when they are lost (or better yet, before they get lost). Women do not have the same physiologic need for a moderate to a long period of time to pass between orgasms (the refractory interval). After a first orgasm, a woman or man becomes very sensitive because of an increase in blood flow. However, after a short time, some women are able to get going again and have another and perhaps multiple orgasms. Men, on the other hand, are able to fall asleep quickly (half-joke).

QUESTION 13
Do women really have a "G-SPOT"?

MAYBE!
Based on research, my opinion is that some women have a prominent, thicker area of nerve endings, blood vessels, and glands/ducts (similar to the male prostate equivalent) near the bladder and muscles in the anterior (front) of the vagina along the course of the urethra (the tube that carries urine from bladder to the outside). However, others do not have such a prominent spot/area. This area has not been consistently confirmed on medical imaging tests, such as an ultrasound or MRI, but that does not mean it is not there.

A bit of history on the subject: the Grafenberg spot or "G-spot" was named by Drs. John Perry and Beverly Whipple for the German obstetrician and gynecologist Dr. Ernst Grafenberg, who wrote about this sensitive area in 1950. Precisely described by some researchers, the G-spot is a sensitive area of tissue that is felt through the anterior (front) wall of the vagina about midway between the back of the pubic bone and the cervix, along the path of the urethra. Potentially the easiest way to find it is when a woman is lying on her back. If 1 or even 2 fingers are placed inside the vagina, with the palm up, using a "come over here" motion, the area or tissue that covers the urethra will apparently begin to swell. Upon first touch of the area, some women will feel like they need to urinate, but if this touch or motion continues for several more seconds, it could turn into a feeling of pleasure. Two sexual positions, the woman on top or vaginal entry from the back or rear, may increase the chance of the penis coming into good contact with the anterior part of the vagina. However, not all women will experience or enjoy stimulation to the area.

Some men enjoy having their prostates stimulated by a partner inserting a lubricated finger or condom-covered lubricated finger into the anus and stroking the area toward the belly. This can produce an orgasm that involves a "bearing-down sensation," which is actually similar to that described in research by some women when they achieve orgasm from G-spot stimulation.

Feel free to experiment a bit with G-spot or prostate stimulation as you and your partner feel comfortable.

QUESTION 14
Do women really fake orgasms? Do most women have regular orgasms from sexual activity and intercourse?

TRUE, FALSE, and FALSE! (sorry folks)
Research continues to show that 50 percent or more of women have faked orgasms. In addition, fewer than 33 percent of women actually have regular orgasms with

their partners, and a similar percentage of women do not have orgasms just from intercourse!

What this really means is there is always room for improvement when it comes to sex. I believe that with help and openness in a relationship those statistics can be improved dramatically. For some couples, just improving communication can increase the odds of an improved sex life.

QUESTION 15
Is the number-one male sexual problem erectile dysfunction? Everyone knows this, right?

FALSE!
The number-one male sexual issue is premature ejaculation, and erectile issues are second to this problem. However, premature ejaculation has numerous safe and wonderful treatment options (see Chapter 10). I am not sure that most people perceive premature ejaculation as a seriously abnormal condition unless it somehow really affects their relationship. Still, options need to be discussed for men and their partners who are concerned.

QUESTION 16
On the news the other night they said that the number-one cause of erectile problems is cardiovascular disease. Is this right?

TRUE!
You really do not need me to tell you why this is the case, do you? Cardiovascular disease has been the number-one killer of men and women in the United States for more than 100 years. Thus, it has also been the biggest killer of erections for more than 100 years! Remember when it was cool to smoke, and smoking was shown in advertising in magazines and all over television? Well, had we advertised that smoking damages all sorts of blood vessels, including those that go to the penis, I wonder if more men would have quit sooner. I remember giving a lecture to some amazing young male athletes, and telling them how many individuals smoking kills around the world annually. I got no reaction. However, when I mentioned that it can "mess up" your penis … well, let's just say I had everyone's attention. You could have heard a pin drop in that room!

QUESTION 17
Do most men with erectile problems have a reduction in testosterone levels?

FALSE!
Many things can affect erections other than testosterone levels, and there are plenty of men with low testosterone who can still have good erections. However,

in some instances, reduced sex drive or penile hardness could be partially due to a low testosterone level. Generally speaking, testosterone replacement therapy (TRT) is not indicated just because a man has a low testosterone level. It may be recommended for a specific person because multiple symptoms of aging are caused by a low testosterone level, and getting TRT would have more benefits as compared to risks. Research is showing that there are a lot of men with low testosterone who function just fine in the bedroom and in other aspects of life.

QUESTION 18
I've heard that most erectile problems are caused by some mental condition or distress. Is this true?

FALSE.
Interestingly, only a decade or two ago it was thought that most cases of erectile dysfunction involved psychological or mental factors, but now we know that this is false. About 80 percent of all cases are due to an "organic" cause (underlying physical medical condition) or "mixed" causes (a combination of psychological and organic). Fewer than 20 percent of cases are thought to be purely psychological in nature.

QUESTION 19
Can high blood sugar levels cause erectile problems? What about lack of sleep and weight gain?

TRUE, TRUE, and TRUE.
High levels of insulin from overly high blood sugar actually creates changes in parts of the sympathetic nervous system that send signals, making it difficult to get an erection, and we need some input from the other part of the nervous system (para-sympathetic) to achieve an adequate erection. In other words, high levels of insulin like to turn the lights in the room on even when you hit the "lights off" switch. Also, high insulin levels cause blood vessels to constrict and reduce blood flow to the penis.

Fewer than 7 hours of sleep a night increases the secretion of endothelin-1, a compound in the body that is actually a powerful blood vessel constricting agent in both men and women. The result is that less blood gets to the sexual organs, possibly contributing to sexual dysfunction. Less sleep also causes an almost immediate (within 1 week) 10 to 15 percent reduction in your daily testosterone levels, which thankfully can be restored back to normal with regular sleep.

A sleep condition, obstructive sleep apnea (OSA), which causes a person to awaken many times a night due to slight breathing interruptions, can result in decreases in other important compounds (not just testosterone) that are needed in higher amounts to cause erections.

QUESTION 20
Are prescription and over-the-counter "man-only prostate" or "hair pills" likely to mess with my sex life?

TRUE!
As mentioned earlier, healthy lifestyle changes improve your sex life, but trying to solve lots of problems with "man pills" can mess up your sex life. For example, what do the best-selling prescription pills for hair loss (finasteride and dutasteride) and prostate enlargement (finasteride, dutasteride, and alpha-blockers) have in common? Answer: Erectile/sexual dysfunction and a loss of sex drive in some men!

Ouch! This is not what we want to hear! We want more hair, but it comes with the potential for less sex? We want smaller prostates, and to pee like we did when we were 15 years old, but this may also reduce our sex drive? Some prostate enlargement pills that do not shrink the prostate can relax the prostate and cause a retrograde ejaculation (in as many as 30 percent of men). When this happens, semen does not leave the body but rather is forced into the urinary bladder, resulting in a "dry orgasm." Some doctors feel that this is no big deal, but others realize that it can impact fertility.

Some prostate enlargement drugs reports these side effects in their handout:
Retrograde ejaculation
Dizziness
Diarrhea
Orthostatic hypotension
Headache
Nasal issues such as congestion

The bottom line is if you are having any of these side effects from your prescription drugs, ask your doctor about switching to one that may have fewer problems, while still working. Or talk with your doctor about coming off these drugs or switching the dosage. They may be great drugs, but perhaps not for everyone.

Over-the-counter pills do not get a free ride. In fact, one of the most common over-the-counter hair tonics and prostate enlargement pills contains saw palmetto, which when taken at a high enough dosage can slightly mimic the side effects of the prescription pills. This means it can result in fewer erections and a less satisfying sex life! Again, as with the prescription options, changing dose or taking other products are all possibilities if you experience this side effect.

To be fair, some men have such bad prostate problems that when an over-the-counter or prescription pill helps them empty their bladder better, they are better able to have and enjoy sex. However, these are the men with the really, really bad prostate issues (the exception, not the rule).

Question 21
Are there other over-the-counter and prescription pills that can impact my sex life?

TRUE!
Approximately, 25 percent of the cases of erectile dysfunction can be linked to prescription and over-the-counter (OTC) medications! WOW! Read that sentence again because that is a big number! SOME medicines (not all of them) in the following categories can cause problems:

Acid reflux drugs (H2 blockers, such as cimetidine and ranitidine)
Alcohol in excess
Antianxiety drugs
Anticholinergics
Anticonvulsants
Antidepressants (30 to 70 percent of men and women experience sexual problems while taking these drugs, which can contribute to poor compliance rates)
Antipsychotics
Blood pressure medications
Cardiac drugs
Cholesterol-lowering drugs
Cocaine (also can kill you, which does not help your sex life)
Diuretics
Marijuana (more carcinogens compared to tobacco, so it can kill you, which does not help your sex life)
Over-the-counter and prescription pain medications (NSAIDs)
Over-the-counter antihistamines, including those that prevent motion sickness
Steroids (especially anabolic steroids used by some athletes)
Tobacco (also can kill you, which does not help your sex life)

Of course we are not advocating that you stop taking drugs that your doctor has prescribed, but it is always a good practice to discuss all possible side effects with your doctor before you begin a new medication (prescription or over-the-counter). However, generally speaking, when it comes to medications and sex, "less is more."

QUESTION 22
Is it true that alcohol in small amounts reduces inhibitions and increases blood flow to the penis?

TRUE!
A small amount of alcohol (1 to 2 drinks maximum) increases the release of nitric oxide in the blood vessels, which slightly opens up more blood flow to the penis.

However, alcohol in excess is a sleep inducer and a sedative, and it may impede your ability to get or sustain an erection. You'll never see this mentioned in beer and alcohol commercials, I'm sure, because it might reduce excessive use of their product when we all choose our love life over intoxication.

QUESTION 23
Can riding a bike cause erectile dysfunction? How about horseback riding?

MAYBE and MAYBE.
However, I would not lose sleep over this. You can purchase a well-fitted bike that makes riding easier on the delicate areas; for example, one with handlebar height that is slightly lower than the bike seat. You can improve your technique, and get a bike (road bike over a mountain bike for some) and bike seat that does not put as much pressure on your perineum (the area between the anus and testicles). Ask your doctor or bike dealer about all of these issues.

It is possible that perineal compression can occur from bike riding. It can lead to blood flow, cellular, and neurologic issues that can increase the risk of erectile problems. Female cyclists could arguably also run the risk of sexual dysfunction issues. However, the risk is small, and bike riding is such a great way to promote cardiovascular health that it can more often reduce the risk of erectile dysfunction.

What about horses? A Texas study found that a "saddle-horn injury of the pelvis," which occurs when a horse rider is thrown into the air and falls back with the perineum hitting the saddle or saddle horn (Ouch!), could cause erectile dysfunction. However, horseback riding can be therapeutic and relaxing, which could improve your mental health, in turn improving your sexual health. Perhaps this is why another study from Minnesota (bet they ride less aggressively than the Texas folk) found no relationship between horseback riders and sexual issues, and a possible reduction in one urinary condition (stress incontinence) in women.

QUESTION 24
Will prescription erectile dysfunction drugs increase sex drive and increase the risk of infidelity?

FALSE and FALSE!
The commercials make it sound so easy ... pop a pill and you will want to do it all night long! Wrong! The prescription drugs definitely are not aphrodisiacs, and they do not make you want to use the equipment significantly more than usual.

They simply make the equipment work better when you do use it.

Individuals interested in increasing sex drive (libido) often consider other treatments more effective for that purpose, such as testosterone replacement therapy (TRT) and/or a male enhancement product (safety and purity are important considerations here), since desire is just as important as making the equipment work better. Some might argue that if your equipment is working better, then your desire for sex will naturally increase. This is true for some men and not true for many other men.

The bottom line is that the United States Food and Drug Administration (FDA) never allows any of the prescription pill companies to claim that they increase sex drive because their research studies did not show a benefit in this area.

The other issue sometimes discussed is whether prescription pills for erectile dysfunction increase the occurrence of infidelity. If men stray, it is simply a moral choice and not the fault of any pill. In fact, relationship issues or problems are listed as the number-one reason for infidelity (not the little blue pill or any other pill).

Also interesting to note: about 20 to 25 percent of men do not respond to ED pills, and about 50 to 66 percent of individuals quit using the drugs after the first prescription is filled!! Regardless of the reason—price, education, or disappointment—the numbers are significant.

QUESTION 25
I don't have erectile dysfunction, but can I enhance my sexual experience by using prescription pills and devices?

FALSE!
Using prescription pills and devices when you do not have erectile function problems not only could cause side effects that are scary, but, in combination with the wrong medicines, could even reduce your blood pressure so much that you fall, faint, get hurt, or in some rare cases, you can cease to exist. In other words, it would be a really stupid thing to do.

QUESTION 26
If a woman takes Viagra, does it cause different side effects as compared to a man? Does it work just as well?

FALSE and FALSE.
In clinical studies, women who took erectile dysfunction prescription pills experienced the same side effects (headache, nasal congestion, flushing, stomach ache, and visual disturbances) as men. And don't forget the high cost! It is extremely unlikely

that Viagra will ever get approved for women because in studies it never worked significantly better than a placebo for women. Having said that, there are some groups of women who may benefit from these drugs. For example, those who experience sexual dysfunction from antidepressant medications, but, as with men, these drugs do NOT increase sexual desire/libido. Antidepressant medications are notorious for causing sexual problems. In women, they can cause a delayed orgasm and reduced lubrication. In men, they can reduce sexual satisfaction. Talk to your doctor.

QUESTION 27
Can testosterone also improve sexual function in women?

MAYBE—with a catch!
Testosterone appears to help some postmenopausal women (or premenopausal women who are producing very little estrogen and/or testosterone) with sexual function and increased sex drive, but there are short-term and long-term safety concerns that need to be addressed. I am not sure whether the women who are prescribed testosterone by their doctors realize that it can permanently deepen the voice, enlarge the clitoris, or cause acne. A woman who considers taking testosterone should be sure that she understands clearly the possible benefits and all the risks, including long-term risks (cancer?). Discuss it carefully with your doctor.

It is worth noting that DHEA supplements in large amounts (hundreds of milligrams a day) can also cause a testosterone increase in some women. It may be toxic to the liver and make cholesterol levels worse. Be sure to talk to a specialist!

Worth mentioning here is that men on steroids also have developed some female features and some serious sexual problems. Consider it carefully with your doctor!

Question 28
Does size matter and will male enhancement pills increase my size?

FALSE (generally speaking) and FALSE!
Hardness is what really matters! Research study after research study, questioning women of all ages, continue to support this fact. If you have a long piece of equipment, well, good for you! However, if that equipment is not really hard, regardless of the size, then this is not so good. Harder and wider equipment provides partners with the stimulation of the clitoral and other areas and the friction needed for sexual pleasure.

A good male-enhancement product, one that focuses on ingredient purity and safety, "maximizes your size" or simply helps to "make you the size you were supposed to be." It does not suddenly and magically make a 6-inch erect penis become an 8-inch penis. "Maximizing your size" is another way of expressing HARDNESS, because if you become hard as possible, then this is naturally maximizing the width and length of your penis. That maximizing helps to increase the chances of a very good sexual experience.

QUESTION 29
Can cold water really shrink a penis?

TRUE!
Cold water reduces the length and width (temporarily) or contracts the penis a bit closer to the abdomen. If you visualize a frightened turtle, you get what I mean. As the penis is contracted in, the higher abdominal core body temperature can warm and save the penis! That it comes with its own survival plan shows you how important this piece of equipment really is. The next time you get called out for "shrinkage," just be strong and tell everyone around you that it is really small now so that it can be really massive when it is called upon for duty! I think you get the idea.

QUESTION 30
Does weight and/or waist loss increase the size of your penis?

TRUE!
In fact, studies show that, as a man gains weight, the excess abdominal tissue begins to pull or retract the penis in toward the abdomen, exposing less of the length of the penis. It is possible that 10 to 15 pounds of weight loss can give a man an extra half-inch of exposed penis length!

QUESTION 31
Is sex in the shower or bathtub dangerous?

FALSE!
Unless you like something really freaky, sex in the shower is generally healthy and safe. It does sometimes have its challenges, though. Lubrication may be a concern because the warm water can have a drying impact for women, and remaining stimulated enough to maintain an erection in a really hot or cold shower is not easy for men. So being turned on or aroused before you get in the shower would be a good idea. Otherwise, using a silicone-based lubricant is a good idea for the shower because it repels water.

QUESTION 32
Oysters and lots of other foods are aphrodisiacs, right?

FALSE!
Oysters, especially raw ones, are not an aphrodisiac. In fact, if you end up getting diarrhea or hepatitis A from eating a contaminated oyster, it can be a real sexual

turn-off. (However, I do love oysters with some hot sauce and lemon juice, which just might kill some microorganisms and improve taste.)

The truth is that oysters are one of the best dietary sources of zinc—one oyster provides more than the recommended daily allowance for zinc. There was some research done a long time ago that suggested that zinc helps to increase the uptake of testosterone into the prostate, and perhaps this is the reason that they were thought to enhance sex drive. However, recent research suggests that men and women are getting too much dietary zinc. In fact, high zinc levels could perhaps increase prostate size in older men over the long term and arguably could increase the risk of sexual dysfunction due to an enlarged prostate.

Bottom line, eat oysters for the taste, and not because you think it will make you or your partner into some kind of sexual dynamo! There is little or no scientific evidence to support the existence of aphrodisiac properties in the other foods on the list that follows, either, but I suppose there is no harm in conducting your own research.

Anise
Asparagus
Cayenne
Chocolate
Coffee
Cucumbers
Mustard
Parsley

Pistachio nuts: Interestingly, a recent small study showed an increase in erectile function within 3 weeks when consuming these nuts daily (see Chapter 2 for other tips on sexual function).

Watermelon: Although the rind contains L-citrulline, which in some individuals could improve sexual health, who eats the rind?

QUESTION 33
I hear that more housework can equal more sex, that headaches and stress can equal more sex, and that even colds and flu can equal more sex. Is this true?

TRUE! TRUE! TRUE! (in theory, at least)
You think that I am joking? Nope! In relationships where one partner (man or woman) does most or all of the household chores, research suggests that sharing the chore burden more evenly can be perceived as an aphrodisiac by the individual

who was previously responsible for all the work. Did I run home and do all the laundry after reading this study? You bet!

Regarding the link between headaches and sex, please let your partner know that sex and orgasms help to release a variety of chemicals, including oxytocin, that cause relaxation, reduces stress, improves mood, and ultimately helps to produce endorphins that are naturally produced painkillers. These same compounds are responsible for what is called "runners' high." It follows that one good way to fight pain, such as a headache, or to reduce stress is to have good sex. In a perfect world, an individual who was overworked or had a headache should want to have sex for selfish reasons!

By the way, recent research suggests that taking too many over-the-counter prescription painkillers can kill your sex life and increases the risk for sexual dysfunction. What does all this mean? Better to have sex solve your pain problems if you can get away with it comfortably!

You are wondering about the colds, aren't you? Several studies have found that frequent sexual activity potentially increases the level of an antibody in the human body, immunoglobulin A, which is secreted to fight infections when you are ill. So, theoretically speaking, if you have an infection such as a cold or flu, you might make it part of the healing process to engage in good sexual activity with your partner. We'll see if this practice catches on as the idea of being sneezed on during sex isn't really appealing.

QUESTION 34
There are so many reasons that sexual problems can occur. How do I know where to go for help?

While it is true that there are many possible causes for sexual problems, it is also true that there are many resources available to help you.

There are sexual abnormalities of desire that can be due to a change in mental health, certain nervous system conditions, hormonal changes, medications, etc. There are erectile dysfunction issues that can be caused by mental health changes, medications, diseases, hormonal changes, blood vessel issues, neuro-logic problems, and even diseases or problems with the penis itself. There are ejaculation problems that can occur for multiple reasons, such as mental health changes, medical conditions, medications, hormones, neurologic changes, etc. There are problems with ORGASM that can be due to medications, mental health, neurologic diseases, etc. There are structural or anatomical penile issues from a variety of causes.

These problems can occur by themselves or in combination, but the real bottom line is that SEXUAL HEALTH is sometimes dismissed as easy to achieve, when in reality it can be quite complex. In many cases individuals benefit from working with a specialist who practices in these areas. Please do not hesitate to contact a health-care professional if you believe you are having any issues.

There are more options available for men and women (lifestyle changes, supplements, prescriptions, procedures, counseling, etc.) compared to any other time in medical history! You have to ask for help, which is actually the toughest step. This book is intended to make you feel more comfortable in finding what you need to solve or even prevent a future problem.

If you do seek medical help, be sure to find a doctor who makes you feel comfortable as you discuss personal issues. My health-care mantra is "LIFE IS TOO SHORT TO HAVE A BAD DOCTOR," but "LIFE IS GOOD WHEN YOU HAVE A GOOD DOCTOR!" I hope that this book really empowers you to live life to its fullest, and a healthy sexual life helps you reach this goal!

CHAPTER 2

Dr. Moyad's Sexual Enhancement Diet for Men and Women

Fact: The European Urologic Association (EAU) guidelines on treating male sexual dysfunction states: "Lifestyle changes and risk factor modification must precede or accompany ED treatment."

What does that mean? It is a grade-A recommendation, which is of the highest level. It means that the EAU recognizes the importance of changing lifestyle and diet factors as part of a treatment plan for erectile dysfunction. Interesting ... let's explore this a bit more.

Theoretically speaking, there is a proven sexual enhancement diet. It is known as the "Heart-Healthy Diet." Anything that promotes heart health in diet or activity also promotes penis health and sexual health in women. Let me emphasize that a second time ... if a diet or activity is good for your heart, it is also good for your sexual health, your libido, your erectile health, your orgasm health, and your intercourse satisfaction.

Yes, it is that simple, but unfortunately not always that easy to follow. Compliance rates on these multiple dietary and lifestyle changes run less than 5 percent in the United States alone!

Let's check out the research on the topic. The Mediterranean diet has the most scientific research published in medical journals on improving sexual health. (This does not mean that other heart-healthy diets do not provide the same benefits; it just means that the Mediterranean diet is supported by the most published papers on improving sexual health.)

So, what was involved in the Mediterranean diet used in these studies? Let's review the components of the diet with a simple checklist.

Dietary Component	Score 1 point for each question answered "yes," and 0 points for a "no" answer
Alcohol (any type)—2 drinks a day or fewer for men and 1 drink or fewer for women	
Fat intake—focused on healthy fats, (canola, olive, safflower oil, etc.), mostly items high in monounsaturated and polyunsaturated fats and low in saturated fats	
Fish—at least 2 or more servings per week of a fatty, oily fish high in omega-3 fatty acids	
Fruit—4 or more servings a day	
Legumes/beans—2 or more servings a week	
Lean meat—1 or fewer servings a day, with minimal intake of red or processed meat	
Nuts and seeds—2 or more servings a week	
Vegetables (other than potatoes)— 4 or more servings a day	
Whole grains (for example, whole/multigrain and whole wheat foods with high amount of fiber and protein)—2 or more servings a day	
TOTAL SCORE	

Note: Traditional Mediterranean diets also allow moderate intakes of dairy, such as cheese, milk, and yogurt. They also involve regular moderate physical activity and social time and social interaction among friends and family members.

Just review the checklist, and add up your points. The Mediterranean diet adherence study has been published all over the world as a general and fast way to determine if someone is following a healthy lifestyle, especially in terms of diet. Individuals with scores of 6 or more on the checklist were closer to following the guidelines of this diet and getting benefits from it as compared to those with scores of 4 or less. There are numerous versions of the checklist, but I have modified it to make it a little more understandable and easy to follow. So, how did you stack up? Is there room for improvement in your diet or exercise plan? Read on...

Let's review Dr. Moyad's Top 8 Recommendations for Sexual Health!

RECOMMENDATION #1

Follow probability-based education, which means you should know your risk factors for diseases and reduce your greatest risk factors first. You should know your fasting cholesterol numbers, your blood pressure values, and other cardiovascular markers, as well as your other "health numbers."

Cholesterol Numbers

Total Cholesterol—lower is better

<160 mg/dL (<4.1 mmol/L)	Ideal or optimal
160–200 mg/dL (4.14–5.16 mmol/L)	Desirable or not bad
200–239 mg/dL (5.16–6.19 mmol/L)	Borderline high
≥240 mg/dL (≥6.22 mmol/L)	High

LDL ("bad cholesterol")—lower is better.

70 mg/dL (<1.81 mmol/L)
May be ideal for some high-risk individuals (those who have already experienced a cardiovascular event or are considered high risk for a cardiovascular event). However, 10 years from now this may be the new normal level. Personally, I believe everyone should try to achieve this level.

<100 mg/dL (<2.59 mmol/L)	Ideal or optimal for most individuals (Dr. Moyad thinks everyone should have an LDL less than 100 right now.)
100–129 mg/dL (2.59–3.34 mmol/L)	Near ideal or optimal/above optimal (feels better ... almost there)

130–159 mg/dL (3.37–4.12 mmol/L)	Borderline high (I do not like this number.)
160–189 mg/dL (4.14–4.90 mmol/L)	High (Fix this problem now.)
≥190 mg/dL (≥4.92 mmol/L)	Very high (Fix this problem immediately.)

HDL ("good cholesterol")—higher is better

≥60 mg/dL (≥1.55 mmol/L)	High or ideal (Awesome or A+)
40–59 mg/dL (1.04–1.53 mmol/L)	Less than ideal (But normal … not bad.)
<40 mg/dL (<1.04 mmol/L)	Too low (Not good—needs work ASAP.)

Triglycerides (fat in the blood)—lower is better.

<100 mg/dL (<1.13 mmol/L)	Dr. Moyad thinks everyone should be below 100!
101–149 mg/dL (1.13–1.69 mmol/L)	Normal (I guess.)
150–199 mg/dL (1.70–2.25 mmol/L)	Borderline high (Reduce this ASAP.)
200–499 mg/dL (2.26–5.64 mmol/L)	High (Reduce this now.)
≥500 mg/dL (≥5.65 mmol/L)	Too high (Do I need to say anything else?)

hs-CRP Numbers

Your hs-CRP score (high-sensitivity C-reactive protein, also known as "cardiac CRP") is a measure of low-grade inflammation that may be occurring in your cardiovascular system. There are other inflammatory markers, but these should be discussed with your doctor. Higher levels may be associated with a higher risk. Some doctors like this test because it is cheap and it has received preliminary testing in women as well as men. I love this test for everyone! Do not confuse this test with a basic CRP test (without the letters hs in front of it), because the basic CRP test is not as sensitive. Ask your doctor if this is a test you should have.

Blood Pressure (Systolic/Diastolic)	What does this mean?
Less than 120/80 mm Hg	Normal, low risk
120–139/80–89 mm Hg	Pre-hypertensive (moderately high or pre-high blood pressure), moderate risk
140/90 mm Hg or greater	Hypertensive (high blood pressure), high risk

RECOMMENDATION #2

Your body mass index (BMI), and more importantly your waist circumference (WC) measurement, should become a standard part your clinical record. Lower is better!

BMI	What does this mean?
Less than 25	Normal weight
25 to 29	Overweight
30 or more	Obese
Waist circumference	**What does this mean?**
Less than 35 inches (or 89 centimeters) in MEN	Normal
35 to 39 inches (or 89 to 100 centimeters) in MEN	Overweight
40 or more inches (101 or more centimeters) in MEN	Obese
Less than 32.5 inches (or 83 centimeters) in WOMEN	Normal
32.5 to 36 inches (or 83 to 93 centimeters) in WOMEN	Overweight
37 or more inches (94 or more centimeters) in WOMEN	Obese

RECOMMENDATION #3

Emphasize fitness and overall health by getting approximately 30 to 60 minutes of physical activity a day or more, depending on individual need. Lift weights or perform resistance exercises several times per week. Aerobic and resistance exercise should be emphasized equally; one is not more vital than the other.

Studies show that exercise significantly reduces your risk of developing many health conditions. Check out the chart that follows, and you'll get up and start moving for sure!

Reduction in Risk with Regular Exercise

Alzheimer's disease & some other types of dementia	30–40 percent
Breast cancer	20–30 percent
Colon cancer	30–50 percent
Depression	25–50 percent
Erectile dysfunction (ED)	25–50 percent
Female sexual dysfunction (FSD)	25–50 percent
Heart disease (all types of CVD)	40–50 percent
Osteoporosis	40–50 percent
Parkinson's disease	unknown percentage, but reduces the risk
Premature death (sudden death)	30–50 percent
Prostate cancer, prostatitis, prostate enlargement	25–50 percent
Stroke	30–50 percent
Type II diabetes	30–40 percent

Weightlifting Benefits (2 times per week)

Bone health—Stimulates bone growth and reduces the risk of osteoporosis, and improves strength, balance, and coordination, which reduces the risk of falls and bone fracture.

Cardiovascular health—Exercises the heart muscle. (Note: If you have a heart condition like an aortic aneurysm or dissection, many doctors do not want you to lift weights … I agree.)

Energy levels/Mood/Fatigue—Reduces fatigue by as much as 50 percent in some studies. Improves energy levels by increasing the efficiency of the body in producing energy. All of this means an increased chance of improved mood during the entire day!

Joint health—Weightlifting and strength training cause muscles to grow and become stronger, reducing the amount of weight or pressure on joints, and may improve or prevent osteoarthritic problems.

Muscle health—We all know this, but increasing lean muscle mass helps not only to improve overall strength but also to make you burn calories more effectively.

Neurologic health—Improves balance and increases insulin sensitivity of the body so it lowers blood glucose and allows the electrical wiring of the body to work more effectively.

Blood sugar health/diabetes—Improves the body's ability to maintain a normal sugar level by increasing the sensitivity of your cells to insulin, so it can reduce your risk of diabetes or improve your diabetes!

Waist & weight loss—Perhaps the most effective way to lose waist and weight, because more lean muscle mass means a faster metabolism and improved body appearance or tone!

RECOMMENDATION #4

Reduce unhealthy dietary fat intake and be encouraged to increase the consumption of healthy fats. In other words, saturated fat, trans-fatty acids, and even dietary cholesterol should be reduced and replaced by more healthy types of monounsaturated or polyunsaturated fat (omega-3 fatty acids).

Specific type of dietary fat	Where it is commonly found?	Good or bad fat? Impact on cholesterol?
Monounsaturated fat	Healthy cooking oils (canola, olive, safflower), nuts	Good Lowers LDL Increases HDL
Polyunsaturated fat (includes omega-3 fatty acids)	Healthy cooking oils (canola, soybean), flaxseed, fish, nuts, soybeans	Good Lowers LDL Increases HDL
Saturated fat (also known as hydrogenated fat)	Non-lean meat, high-fat dairy, some fast food	Mostly bad (only because it is associated with high caloric intake). Increases LDL Increases HDL
Trans fat (also known as partially hydrogenated fat)	Some margarines, fast food, snack foods, deep-fried foods	Bad Increases LDL Lowers HDL

If you reduce your intake of saturated fat, in general you lower your intake of calories, too. As an example, let's look at whole milk, 2 percent, 1 percent, and skim milk, and tell me what you notice.

Type of milk	Saturated Fat/Serving	Calories/Serving
Almond milk	0 grams	40–60
Soy milk	0 grams	80–100
Skim milk	0 grams	80
1% milk	1.5 grams	100
2% milk	3 grams	120
Whole milk	5 grams	150

If you work to reduce your intake of saturated fats, you'll get an added bonus of reducing your calories—two health benefits in one!

RECOMMENDATION #5

Consume a diversity of low-cost fruits and vegetables and not high-caloric, expensive, and high-antioxidant exotic juices. Dietary supplements that claim to substitute for fruit and vegetable consumption are not recommended. Also, never forget that regular alcohol consumption is one of the best ways to gain weight!

Check out the following chart of beverage caloric contents and you'll see how you can make a smarter choice by selecting lower-calorie beverages.

Beverage	Calories/serving
Mixed fruit smoothie	200–250
Acai juice	150–200
Grape juice	170–180
Pomegranate juice	140–160
Pineapple juice or cherry juice	130–150
Orange, grapefruit, apple juices, or lemonade	100–120
Beer/wine/hard liquor	100–150
Watermelon juice	100–110
Cola and other soft drinks	100
Skim or soy milk	80–100
Carrot juice	70–80
Cranberry juice	70–80
Light beer	70–80
Blueberry juice	50–60

Gatorade® sports drink	50
Tomato juice or mixed vegetable tomato-based juice	50
Coffee (with fat-free milk to cream)	5–50
Tea (black, green, Oolong)	0–5
Diet soft drink	0
Water	0

RECOMMENDATION #6

Consume more total (soluble and insoluble) dietary fiber (20–30 grams/day) from food for overall health advantages. One-third of a cup of bran cereal with flaxseed or chia seed and some fruit provides approximately 20 grams of fiber and gives you a good start to the day. The following list provides a sampling of foods that are both high in fiber and delicious. Consider adding more of them to your diet.

Top Sources of Dietary Fiber	Grams of Fiber
Vegetables	
Artichoke (1 whole, cooked)	10
Artichoke hearts (1 cup)	7
Parsnips (1 cup)	5.5
Broccoli (1 cup)	4.5
Brussels sprouts (1 cup)	4.5
Legumes and Beans	
Cranberry beans (2/3 cup)	12
Baked beans (1/2 cup)	9
Kidney beans (1/2 cup)	7–8
Split peas (1/2 cup)	6.7
Navy beans (1/2 cup)	6
Grains and Cereals	
Wheat-bran cereal (All-Bran, FiberOne) (1/3 cup)	10–14
Oatmeal (3/4 cup)	4–5
Bran Chex cereal (2/3 cup)	4.5
Raisin bran–type cereals	4
Spaghetti (whole wheat) (1/2 cup cooked)	4–6
Nuts and Seeds	
Flaxseed (golden/brown) (2 Tbsp.)	4–6
Chestnuts (10 roasted kernels)	4–5
Chia seeds (1 Tbsp.)	4–5
Almonds (5 nuts)	3–4
Sunflower seeds (1 oz.)	3–4

RECOMMENDATION #7

Increase your weekly intake of a variety of canned, broiled, baked, and even raw or smoked fish in your diet. Avoid fish that is fried and certain types of fish that tend to be high in mercury. Other healthy sources of omega-3 fatty acids (for example, nuts and healthy plant cooking oils) are also encouraged. As you'll see from the list that follows, the amount of omega-3 varies greatly in different kinds of fish. Try to pick those from the list with the highest level of omega-3 that are also lower in mercury.

Fish	Total Omega-3 Amount
Anchovy*	1,165 mg
Catfish (farmed)	250 mg
Catfish (wild)	350 mg
Clams	240 mg
Cod (Atlantic)	285 mg
Cod (Pacific)	435 mg
Crab (Alaskan king)	350 mg
Fish sandwich (fast food)	335 mg
Fish sticks (frozen)	195 mg
Flounder/Sole	500 mg
Halibut	740 mg(high in mercury)
Haddock	200 mg
Herring* (Atlantic or Pacific)	1,710 mg
King mackerel	620 mg (high in mercury)
Lobster	70 mg
Mackerel (Atlantic)*	1,060 mg
Mahimahi	220 mg
Mussels	665 mg
Oysters (Eastern, farmed, Pacific)	585 mg
Pollock (Alaskan)	280 mg
Salmon (farmed)*	1,775 mg +
Salmon (wild)*	1,775 mg (high in vitamin D3)
Sardines*	555 mg
Scallops	310 mg
Shrimp	265 mg
Shark	585 mg (high in mercury)
Snapper	545 mg
Swordfish	870 mg (high in mercury)
Tilapia	100-150 mg
Tilefish or golden bass	1,360 mg (high in mercury)
Trout* (rainbow, farmed, or wild)	580–800 mg

Tuna (fresh)	900 mg (moderate to high in mercury)
Tuna (light, skipjack)	230 mg
Tuna (white, albacore)	735 mg (high in mercury)
Whitefish (Great Lakes)	1,350 mg

*Fish in bold are moderate in their level of mercury, practical, and generally safe to eat to get your recommended daily allowance of fish oil for heart health. It's okay to deviate several times a month, for example by eating halibut or regular tuna, because they are high in omega-3, and the benefits of eating fish regularly usually outweigh the concern over mercury toxicity.

RECOMMENDATION #8
Please constantly and consistently emphasize heart-healthy lifestyle recommendations (numbers 1–7) because the best research shows that these recommendations precisely mirror the most effective sexual health advice tips that you can follow. Remember, the sum total of the positive health practices individuals can carry out in moderation has the highest probability of impacting male sexual and overall health much more than doing just one or two lifestyle changes to the extreme.

To end this chapter, I've included my favorite self-help quiz. These moderate lifestyle changes can greatly reduce the risk of a first cardiovascular event, and they just might enhance your sex life as well! Check it out and see how you score.

DR. MOYAD'S HEART-HEALTHY, SEX-HEALTHY QUIZ

Test your health IQ!
Circle the answer to each question.

1. I currently smoke.
A. Yes (–10 points, yes, that is a minus)
B. No (0 points)

2. What is your LDL (bad cholesterol) untreated or treated with medication?
A. Less than 100 mg/dl or 2.59 mmol/L (4 points)
B. 100–129 mg/dl or 2.59–3.34 mmol/L (3 points)
C. 130–159 mg/dl or 3.37–4.12 mmol/L (2 points)
D. 160–189 mg/dl or 4.14–4.90 mmol/L (1 point)
E. 190 mg/dl or 4.92 mmol/L and above (0 points)
F. Do not know the answer (–1 point)

3. What is your HDL (good cholesterol) untreated or treated with medication?
A. 60 mg/dl or 1.55 mmol/L and above (4 points)
B. 50–59 mg/dl or 1.29–1.53 mmol/L (3 points)
C. 40–49 mg/dl or 1.04–1.27 mmol/L (2 points)
D. 35–39 mg/dl or 0.91–1.01 mmol/L (1 point)
E. Below 35 mg/dl or 0.91 mmol/L (0 points)
F. Do not know the answer (–1 point)

4. What is your triglyceride number untreated or treated with medication?
A. Less than 100 mg/dl or 1.13 mmol/L (4 points)
B. 100–149 mg/dl or 1.13–1.68 mmol/L (3 points)
C. 150–199 mg/dl or 1.70–2.25 mmol/L (2 points)
D. 200–499 mg/dl or 2.26–5.64 mmol/L (1 point)
E. 500 mg/dl or 5.65 mmol/L and above (0 points)
F. Do not know the answer (–1 point)

5. Your hs-CRP (high sensitivity C-Reactive protein) blood level is:
A. Normal (2 points)
B. Abnormal (1 point)
C. I don't know/have not had this tested (–1)

6. You fasting blood glucose level is:
A. Normal (2 points)
B. Abnormal (1 point)
C. I don't know/have not had this tested (–1)

7. Your blood pressure untreated or treated is:
A. Less than 120/80 mmHg (4 points)
B. 120–139 and/or 80–89 mmHg (3 points)
C. 140 or higher and/or 90 mmHg or higher (2 points)
D. Do not know (1 point)

8. Aerobic exercise and/or weight-lifting/resistance exercise
A. I exercise an average of 30 minutes a day and lift weights/do resistance exercises 2 to 3 times a week. (4 points)
B. I exercise an average of 30 minutes a day, but I do not lift weights/do resistance exercises on a regular basis. (3 points)
C. I lift weights/do resistance exercises regularly, but do not do regular aerobic exercise (2 points).
D. I do not exercise or lift weights/do resistance exercises regularly (1 point).
E. I do not have any time to exercise or lift weights/do resistance exercises (0 points)

9. Two types of "healthy" dietary fats are _____ and _____.
A. Monounsaturated and polyunsaturated fat (4 points)
B. Monounsaturated and trans fat (3 points)
C. Polyunsaturated and trans fat (2 points)
D. Saturated and trans fat (1 point)
E. All dietary fat is unhealthy (0 points)

10. How many servings of alcohol do you drink a day?
(1 serving is 12 ounces of beer, 4–6 ounces of wine, or 1.5 ounces of hard liquor)
A. If female 1 or fewer servings/day and if male 2 or fewer servings/day (4 points)
B. If female 2 or fewer servings/day and if male 3 or fewer servings/day (2 points)
C. Any other answer (0 points)

11. How much fiber do you get in your diet per day?
(Insoluble fiber comes from healthy foods, not pills and powders)
A. 20–30 grams a day and mostly insoluble fiber (4 points)
B. 20–30 grams a day and mostly soluble fiber (3 points)
C. 10–20 grams a day and mostly insoluble fiber (2 points)
D. 10–20 grams a day and mostly soluble fiber (1 point)
E. Less than 10 grams a day (0 points)
F. I do not know (–1 point)

12. I get my omega-3 fatty acids mostly from eating:
A. Plant sources and 2–3 servings/week of non-fried, small-to-medium-size oily
   fish such as anchovies, mackerel, salmon, sardines (4 points)
B. Plant sources and 1–2 servings/week of non-fried, small-to-medium-size oily
   fish such as anchovies, mackerel, salmon, sardines (3 points)
C. Plant sources and 0–1 servings/week of non-fried, small-to-medium-size oily
   fish such as anchovies, mackerel, salmon, sardines (2 points)
D. I just take a fish oil pill (1 point)
E. I do not eat fish or a take a fish oil pill (0 points)

13. How many servings of fruits and vegetables do you eat per day?
A. More than 1 serving a day (4 points)
B. Less than 1 serving a day (3 points)
C. A couple of servings a week (2 points)
D. A couple of servings a month (1 point)
E. I do not like fruits or vegetables (0 points)
F. I only eat colorful fruits and veggies because they are the healthiest (–1 point)

14. I like fruits and vegetable juices that:
A. Taste good and have the lowest calories (4 points)
B. Taste good regardless of calories (1 point)
C. Regardless of taste, have the highest concentration of antioxidants (0 points)

15. I like to have sex/make love with my partner at least:
A. Several times a week (1 point)
B. Once a week (1 point)
C. Once every 2 weeks or month (0 points)
D. Not that often (0 points)
E. I do not like to have sex with my partner (–1 point)

16. I average about ___ hours of sleep per night.
A. 7–8 hours (1 point)
B. 5–6 hours (1 point)
C. 3–4 hours (0 points)

17. I get ___ milligrams (mg) of sodium a day from food and beverages.
A. 1,500 mg or less (1 point)
B. 1,501 mg–2,300 mg (1 point)
C. 2,301 mg or more (0 points)

18. My mood and stress level is generally:
A. Excellent, usually very happy (1 point)
B. Very good, usually happy (1 point)
C. Good, moderately happy (1 point)
D. Indifferent, not really happy or sad (0 points)
E. Bad (–1 point)

Now that you've totaled your score, look the quiz over again to see what changes you could make in your routine that might improve your health profile.

For more information on diet and health ...

Dr. Moyad's No BS Health Advice
ISBN: 978-1-58726-256-2
$19.95

www.sprypub.com

CHAPTER 3

Over-the-Counter Sexual Enhancement Solutions

As you listen to the radio or read advertisements, you are immediately struck by what a big business over-the-counter sexual enhancement sales are. The claims are often astounding! However, the reality isn't quite as astounding. The truth is that the FDA has removed over 70 of them from the market. 70! Many are either formulated without the benefit of any research or adulterated with drug-like compounds that can be dangerous to your health. If they do contain a beneficial component, they may also be loaded with ingredients that dilute any potential benefit. For more than a decade, consumers have been left with a choice between ridiculously expensive prescription medications complete with many potential side effects or sketchy supplements making a host of unfounded claims. Yet, I know from the many, many questions I have gotten during presentations and meetings with individuals over my career that both the interest in and the need for a better product exist.

Actually, those many, many compounds that the FDA removed from the market indirectly led to my involvement with the development of the supplement Triverex. I always urge individuals to consider scientific research and purity of ingredients when evaluating any supplement, but I couldn't find a single male enhancement supplement that I felt comfortable recommending. In my work with the Triverex team, I have had the opportunity to review both the research and the assurance of purity on the product components to the point that I am comfortable recommending (and taking) the supplement, along with many other physicians.

However, I believe that you should do your own homework and thoroughly review any supplement that you consider taking. In the following section, I'll help evaluate "the good, the bad, and the ugly" of many compounds used in supplements. You'll also read about a variety of options that should be avoided altogether, or ones that simply have no research to show whether they might work or not.

Quick Thoughts About Dietary Supplements
There are several thoughts that I always use in considering the value of any supplement. These are good tips to help you evaluate a product. If it isn't heart healthy, it isn't worth taking as a supplement for sexual enhancement or any other purpose.

It has to provide some tangible benefit, otherwise forgettaboutit! Natural does not always mean better. Arsenic is a natural product, and you wouldn't take that. Let the research decide if natural is really better for you; otherwise no one has any idea.

Test tube and rat studies should not be the reason you take a supplement unless you are a test tube or a rat. It is a fact that as many as 99 percent of supplements work well in test tubes and rats, but you would be lucky if 1 percent of what worked in test tubes and rats actually work for you. Let human studies and consultation with a trusted health-care professional who knows something about dietary supplements help you decide what to take. The best "expert" in the field of dietary supplements is someone who works full time in that field and who is respected by other recognized health-care professionals. The old analogy about not using a part-time surgeon or part-time mechanic to do your surgery or service your car definitely applies here!

The list that follows includes both over-the-counter supplements and therapies that have been touted to improve sexual health. In each case, I've offered my recommendation on the treatment.

Acupuncture
Recommended: YES!
Acupuncture, meditation, massage, and other therapies that are mentally and physically relaxing can help especially when stress, anxiety, depression or other mental issues are the cause of the problem. They can even possibly reduce pain, which may be the reason for lack of sexual activity. Any type of exercise or procedure that can help you relax could translate into an improvement in your sexual health.

Ashwagandha (Withania somnifera)
Recommended: NO!
Efficacy and safety in humans have not been adequately tested.

Avena sativa pills
Recommended: NO!
Avena sativa is the common oat—also known as wild oats, oat bran, or oat straw—and has been shown to potentially reduce cholesterol and blood pressure in some studies. Heck, it's oats! I heartily recommend it for breakfast. However, some male enhancement product companies offer Avena sativa as a supplement ingredient, perhaps believing that reducing cholesterol levels/blood pressure or changing the male hormone environment may improve sexual function. This might be true if you regularly consume oat bran (good source of fiber), but getting a small quantity from pills is a different story. The use of pills is not supported by human studies. On the practical side, it can take as many as 30 to 60 fiber capsules a day to get

your recommended daily allowance of fiber, so stick with flaxseed, chia seed, fruits and veggies, and breakfast cereals that are high in insoluble fiber.

Catuaba (Erythroxylum catuaba)
Recommended: NO!
Efficacy and safety in humans have not been adequately tested.

Coenzyme Q10
Recommended: MAYBE for Peyronie's Disease
A recent large study found that approximately 300 mg a day of CoQ10 could improve sexual function in men with Peyronie's, which is a condition that can cause uncomfortable curvature of the penis (see chapter 10 for more information). Additionally, this supplement is being tested to reduce a side effect of cholesterol-lowering drugs (muscle discomfort), and there is preliminary research that suggests it may reduce blood pressure in individuals who have hypertension or risk factors for hypertension. Therefore, it should not be a surprise that it will be receiving more research to see if it can improve sexual function.

Cordyceps
Recommended: NO!
Efficacy and safety in humans have not been adequately tested.

Damiana
Recommended: NO!
A complete mess! No legitimate studies and no idea on safety, except that it does contain compounds ("cyanide-like") that could make it toxic. How this substance traditionally used as a tea found its way into certain male enhancement formulas is an unsolved mystery—move over, Big Foot and the Loch Ness Monster.

DHEA
Recommended: NO
This is the craziest supplement for most men! Why? Simply because prescription testosterone does everything that this can do and more, and it is safer and smarter. In higher doses, DHEA can increase estrogen levels in a man as much as it increases testosterone. This happens because DHEA is converted to both testosterone AND estrogen in men. It is an unpredictable process, so some men will make more estrogen and some will make more testosterone. Who would want that?

Also, DHEA is given orally, causing some issues with cholesterol that are never good. In many of the largest dose studies, men who took DHEA had significant drops in their good cholesterol (HDL). This is not heart healthy! Remember the first tip on supplements earlier? If it isn't heart healthy—pass on it! However, there are always very rare exceptions. In a small number of cases (usually for female sexual issues) where an individual has a low DHEA level, taking 25 to 50 mg per day might help a little in the sexual function area after a short period of time. If you think this might apply to you, then ask your doctor about taking a DHEA or DHEA-S blood test to determine your actual level before considering the supplement. Normal levels vary based on your age group so your physician can help you assess your results.

Eleuthero (Eleutherococcus senticosus)

Recommended: NO!
This product is better known as Siberian ginseng, but in reality it is not related to ginseng. Efficacy and safety in humans have not been adequately tested.

Fenugreek (Trigonella foenum-graecum)

Recommended: Needs More Study
Human studies have failed to demonstrate that this herb/spice supplement increases testosterone consistently, which is what it is often advertised to do. In fact, some recent human studies have shown that it may actually reduce testosterone. The funny thing about this product is that it has been around for a long time. Some researchers thought it would reduce cholesterol, which it has not really done, but it may have some blood-thinning effects that cause concern. Gastrointestinal side effects and possible allergic reactions are possible with this product because of some of the allergenic-like compounds that occur naturally in the plant. Fenugreek seeds (not to be confused with the supplement) may slightly reduce cholesterol because they contain fiber, but better fiber sources are readily available.

Folic acid

Recommended: NO WAY!
Also known as vitamin B9, it has no real function in male enhancement. Folic acid's claim to fame is its ability to prevent neural tube defects in babies whose mothers take it during pregnancy, but for men it may just increase the risk of future prostate problems. Excessive long-term intake of supplemental folic acid could increase the risk of abnormal tissue growth (aka cancer). There is no adequate human study to even suggest that it helps men with their sexual health. While some studies show that folic acid can improve sperm count, there are plenty of safer supplements for men that can also do that (CoQ10, L-carnitine, omega-3, etc.).

Ginkgo biloba

Recommended: NO! PARTICULARLY NEVER BEFORE A SURGICAL PROCEDURE.
This herbal product may increase bleeding time, increase the risk of bleeding internally, and create excessive blood thinning in those on blood thinning medications (even aspirin). In some clinical studies, this herbal product or an extract of it was associated with increases in the risk of strokes. The risk of using it regularly

appears to outweigh any potential benefits. The erectile function studies with ginkgo suggest that, if it really helps, it may slightly help some people with sexual problems associated with antidepressant drugs. However, other supplements are safer. Potent blood thinning in a person who does not need more blood thinning should be a cause for concern. Similar to a leak in a hose, thinning the blood too much can allow it to escape out of the circulatory system and into areas where it may be dangerous.

Ginseng
Recommended: YES!
Korean/Panax ginseng may have some efficacy. (Not the Siberia ginseng discussed earlier, which, as you may recall, is not related to true ginseng.) A qualifier to the recommendation is that you need to watch out for quality control issues with ginseng. Be sure that you know that the maker of the supplement you are considering monitors purity and safety of its components. Korean ginseng has over 100 compounds in it, but only a handful of those have evidence that they can improve sexual health. Ginseng can lead to trouble unless you can find a product that has exactly the right research-based compounds for sexual health, in the correct dosage, and is not contaminated with other ingredients.

Horny goat weed (Epimedium sagittatum)
Recommended: MAYBE!
The research on this compound is increasing, but again quality control is a major problem. Be sure that the supplement that you are considering monitors purity and safety of its components. This compound is supposed to help with blood flow.

L-arginine
Recommended: MAYBE from pills, and yes from diet
Arginine is an amino acid that is produced by the body, and L-arginine is one of the 20 most common amino acids. In addition to the amount you produce, you get it from your diet. One of the functions of L-arginine in the body is to produce nitric oxide (NO), an agent that dilates blood vessels and improves blood flow. It definitely is one of the most misunderstood supplements for male health. Some people think that all they need to do is take this supplement, and then they get a Viagra-like impact. Wrong!

In reality, the body is far more efficient itself at converting other internal compounds to nitric oxide than any L-arginine supplement. Also, when you take it in a pill form, L-arginine is rapidly metabolized and degraded by the intestines, and, in fact, the liver gets rid of most of it. The little that does get into the blood does not survive there long. I don't recommend taking mega-doses of a supplement that would be necessary to possibly create a sexual enhancement effect. It makes more sense overall to take another supplement that can cause production of L-arginine naturally and safely in the body, bypassing the digestive process. There is a supplement with arginine and pycnogenol that may help some men, but I would never take these products without being monitored by a medical expert.

It is worth noting that when L-arginine as a pill does reach the blood stream it can cause a rather large drop in blood pressure for a short period, perhaps dangerous in some individuals.

If you remain convinced that L-arginine is a possibility for you, sticking with some of the dietary sources below is a good option.

Food	Arginine Amount (g/100g)
Pine nuts	3,000–4,000
Soy beans	2,000–3,000
Sesame seeds	2,000–3,000
Pumpkin seeds	2,000–3,000
Sunflower seeds	2,000–3,000
Peanut butter	2,000–3,000
Peanuts	2,000–3,000
Almonds	1,500–2,000
Brazil nuts	1,500–2,000
Beef	1,500–2,000

Walnuts	1,500–2,000
Halibut	1,000–1,500
Chicken	1,000–1,500
Hazelnuts	1,000–1,500
Pistachios	500–1,000
Tuna (canned)	1,500
Salmon	1,300
Shrimp	1,300
Parmesan cheese	1,300
Egg Yolk	1,000
Lentils	660
Spinach	325
White bread	300
Rice	175

Note: Basically, seafood, nuts, seeds, lean meats, and dairy, and whey, egg white, and other protein powders are high in L-arginine. However, nuts and seeds have arguably larger amounts of free L-arginine. The free L-arginine may be more effective, some preliminary research suggests that L-arginine competes with another amino acid (L-lysine) in some foods (beef and fish) for utilization. Overall, heart-healthy foods are high in L-arginine!

L-carnitine

Recommended: NO (except for those with Peyronie's disease)

The doses needed are too high, and so is the cost. L-carnitine is a compound that helps to transport other items in the body to create energy and potentially repair some injuries. This is why there has been a lot of research on this supplement as a way to reduce fatigue, to improve sexual function, and to improve Peyronie's disease (a condition that causes curvature of the penis). However, although this supplement has a very good safety record, the first problem is the cost. The next lem is the dosage. It is somewhat similar to L-arginine in terms of amounts needed to potentially get a result. I was never sold on this supplement because the cost and the high dosages needed make it difficult to try for a long period of time. New research suggests that different forms of L-carnitine may be better, but the costs of these newer ones are even higher, and high dosages are still needed. OUCH!

L-citrulline
Recommended: YES! LOVE THIS COMPOUND!
L-citrulline is converted into L-arginine in the human body by the kidneys so it is a safe way to get the L-arginine and nitric oxide you need without the extreme blood pressure changes. In addition, there is now human research published in a major urology journal to suggest that this compound is safe and can produce harder erections! Yes, this is what was actually tested in the study—men experienced harder erections. Also, there is plenty of research to now suggest that L-citrulline can improve athletic workouts and recovery from those workouts. One concern: getting L-citrulline in a pure non-adulterated form may not be easy. Be sure that the maker of any supplement you are considering monitors its components for purity and safety. I would love to be able to recommend a dietary source of L-citrulline, but it is almost impossible to obtain much from foods except for watermelon and watermelon rind.

L-theanine
Recommended: MAYBE, especially for those who have stress and anxiety issues.
In Japan, the amino acid L-theanine has been used in all kinds of foods for decades. Now, research suggests that L-theanine in doses of 100 to 200 mg can help reduce anxiety and stress. However, talk with your doctor, because it could slightly lower blood pressure and heart rate. Still, this supplement and another (GABA) have lately been supported by some interesting anti-stress research that could theoretically help some individuals whose sexual health is impacted by anxiety or stress.

Maca (Lepidium meyenii)
Recommended: YES!
Also called the "pride of Peru," maca is a plant that grows only at higher elevations in the central Peruvian Andes. Most natives of Peru will know what you mean when you ask for maca. In fact, when my wife visited Peru, she walked right into the first store and bought me some maca. It is in reality a root vegetable and belongs to the Brassica family (like broccoli, cabbage, etc.). Maca is the name of the plant Lepidium meyenii, which has compounds in it that appear to improve male and female sexual function, including sex drive. There have been multiple clinical studies with maca. In fact, enough studies have been completed that a summary of clinical studies on sexual function was published

in a reputable medical journal. Maca is supported by the second-largest number of clinical studies in men and women pertaining to sexual function, but certain components in Panax ginseng have the most human data. Other studies suggest that maca could improve fertility. The maca root contains a high concentration of amino acids, iodine, iron, magnesium, and a number of other compounds (macamides) that may improve sexual desire. Maca has NOT been found to raise testosterone or estrogen thus far, which means it probably works through some unidentified central/brain activating mechanism, if it truly works. I definitely think it does something, it appears to have a good safety record, and it is used widely in the Peruvian culture.

Milk thistle
Recommended: NO!
It is embarrassing that this is even in some sexual health supplements.

Muira puama (aka "potency wood"?)
Recommended: NO!
This supplement apparently comes from a small bush in the rain forests of Brazil. The bark and root apparently can do things for you. A few older studies suggested benefits, but the absence of anything new on efficacy or safety is a concern.
And, apparently the primary benefit comes from increasing levels of steroid-like compounds (not proven) such as testosterone. Again, why not just get testosterone replacement therapy if you qualify?

Omega-3 fatty acids (ALA, EPA, DHA...)
Recommended: MAYBE, and may get positive research in the future!
These are heart-healthy compounds that are found in high concentrations in flaxseed, chia seed, and healthy fatty fish. They are a part of the Mediterranean diet that can arguably improve sexual health in men and women.

Pycnogenol
Recommended: MAYBE!
This compound from a French maritime pine bark has been advertised to help all sorts of problems. It has some interesting preliminary data in arthritis treatment, and some data for improving sexual function in combination with L-arginine. However, if you have read the section on L-arginine, then you already know why there is very little more I can say about this supplement.

Red clover
Recommended: NO WAY!
This is a fairly potent plant estrogen supplement that, when taken in high concentrations, can increase your breast size (if you are a man) and may cause liver issues. Its estrogenic qualities explain why some individuals have used this pill for hot

flashes. Why the makers would put this product into a male health pill is beyond me unless they believe that men need to get more in touch with their feminine sides.

Rhodiola (Rhodiola rosea)
Recommended: MAYBE (if stress is the issue).
This is an anti-stress supplement. However, L-theanine or GABA by themselves probably make more sense for stress if your doctor gives the okay (see L-theanine, page 48).

SAM-e
Recommended: MAYBE (if depression or arthritis is an issue).
SAM-e is an interesting supplement. Recent research suggests that it may actually improve the efficacy of some prescription antidepressant drugs, or it may be used by itself for depression or arthritis. Talk to your doctor! If pain or mental health issues are the primary cause of your sexual issues, please ask your doctor if you could add this supplement to your program. St. John's Wort is another antidepressant supplement that sells well, but the problem with this herbal product is quality control. It can increase the metabolism of so many drugs that it actually can reduce their efficacy.

Saw palmetto, pygeum, stinging nettle, beta-sitosterol, and other prostate enlargement supplements
Recommended: NO!
Some of these compounds could help some men with mild prostate enlargement, but among their rare side effects is erectile dysfunction, which is exactly what is found with the prescription drugs that work in a similar fashion. Also, recent research suggests that saw palmetto is not as effective as researchers once believed. So why would an individual purchase any product for male enhancement that has saw palmetto or another prostate enlargement supplement in it? I suppose if a man's prostate enlargement is reducing his sexual function and some prescription and/or over-the-counter product (like beta-sitosterol) helps him urinate better, then it may also slightly help with sexual function. However, that being said, it would make much more sense to make heart-healthy lifestyle changes and take a product that directly helps with sexual health.

Tongkat ali or "Longjack" (Eurycoma longifolia)
Recommended: MAYBE
Many supplements that contain this compound claim that they have the potential to increase testosterone levels—maybe for some men with very low testosterone levels. There is preliminary research that it can improve sexual health, so why not try it? Bear in mind, if you are just looking for a dramatic testosterone increase from this supplement, I believe most of you will be disappointed.

Tribulus terrestris
Recommended: WHY?
Just get a prescription of testosterone. Human studies have failed to demonstrate that this herb increases testosterone, which is what it is advertised to do in many places. Why not cut to the chase and get the real thing (testosterone) if you really need it? Tribulus can act like a diuretic, and it may increase blood pressure.

Vitamin A, B-Complex, C, D, E, etc....
Recommended: NO!
None of these common supplements have ever been shown to improve sexual health. In other words, most of the ingredients in a multivitamin do nothing for you in terms of sexual health except reduce the size of your wallet or purse, if you know what I mean.

Yohimbine
Recommended: NO! Not heart healthy!
Yohimbine comes from the West African Yohimbe tree and can be found as a supplement and as a prescription drug. Whether or not it even works is controversial. However, it is an "alpha-2-adrenoreceptor antagonist," and some of the side effects include: headache, sweating, nausea, dizziness, nervousness/agitation, tremors, sleeplessness, anti-diuresis (can't pee), and elevated blood pressure and heart rate. It cannot be taken by individuals with kidney disease, those on antidepressants or other mood-altering drugs, and some individuals with specific cardiovascular, neurological, and psychological issues. This product is such a disaster in terms of lack of effectiveness and excessive side effects that it should be avoided.

Zinc
Recommended: NO!
For acne, yes, because low doses are needed. However, for sexual enhancement—NEVER! Recent and past evidence has demonstrated that mega doses of zinc (recommended by some boneheaded "experts" at 80 or 100 mg or more per day), especially with individual supplements, has the potential to encourage the growth of prostate conditions from BPH to cancer. It also may increase the risk of urinary tract infections and kidney stones. In fact, in one of the largest studies of zinc supplements (a Harvard study), researchers found a significantly higher risk of advanced prostate cancer in men consuming large intakes of these supplements. Other laboratory and clinical data suggests that larger doses of zinc can inhibit the benefits of some prescription drugs, increase testosterone uptake or levels within the prostate, reduce levels of "good cholesterol" or HDL, and cause immune dysfunction. More research is needed in this area, but in the meantime, I would discourage or recommend immediately discontinuing the intake of larger concentrations of zinc for most individuals until adequate research resolves this controversial issue.

CHAPTER 4

Prescription Penis Pills to the Rescue! Maybe?

Let's jump right into this chapter with some fast facts about erectile dysfunction (ED) drugs ...

FACT #1: Cheaper generic ED drugs are on the way.
The main prescription drugs that are used to treat erectile dysfunction are Viagra, Cialis, and Levitra. Viagra received FDA approval in 1998, followed by Cialis and Levitra in 2003. Expiring patents will mean that cheaper generic prescription ED drugs will be here soon. Get ready for prices to drop faster than an erection placed directly into an ice-fishing hole in Lake Michigan in the middle of January! If you and your partner ever visit Brazil, you should note that Viagra has already lost its patent there!

FACT #2: ED drugs do not cause an erection without sexual stimulation.
Relying solely on prescription penis pills to produce an erection would take longer than it takes for a major airline company to put a real person on the phone to talk to you! There aren't any ED drugs that can initiate an erection without some sexual stimulation.

FACT #3: ED drugs do not increase sexual desire on their own, but when regular exercise is added to the mix, these drugs may do the trick!
ED drugs do not significantly increase sex drive. Instead of making you more excited than you already are about having sex, they make your equipment work better once you are aroused. A dirty magazine or poorly produced porn flick does a better job of increasing your sexual desire than prescription penis pills. However, it is okay that ED drugs improve performance and not desire because the companies that make these drugs never claimed they could improve your libido.

Take note: a recent study demonstrated that men taking these drugs who began to exercise regularly experienced an increase in sex drive. It makes sense for Viagra or another ED drug company to collaborate with a fitness company to promote ED drugs and exercise equipment. Another approach would be for ED drug companies to give loyal customers a treadmill to thank them for paying the high price of their prescription penis pills for so long.

FACT #4: ED drugs work for many men with different causes of ED.
These drugs can help men with all sorts of different causes for their ED. One of the biggest advantages of ED drugs has to be that men with diabetes, mental health issues, prostate problems, spinal cord injuries, neurological conditions, or high blood pressure, and men taking certain medications, such as antidepressants, may qualify for this medication.

An interesting fact: ED drugs require the presence or production in the body of a compound called nitric oxide (NO) for them to be most effective. When men have normal levels of testosterone, NO levels tend to be better. Research has demonstrated that some dietary supplements can increase NO levels. It is possible, and may even be helpful, to use a quality-controlled supplement with ED drugs. Numerous doctors and many men have tried combining ED drugs, supplements, and/or testosterone replacement therapy.

FACT #5: ED drugs can significantly reduce your blood pressure, and that drop is not always a good thing.
When a man is taking 100 mg of Viagra, the average systolic blood pressure drop is about 8.5 points, and the average diastolic blood pressure drop is 5.5 points. Because prescription nitrate medications cause blood pressure to drop, they should not be combined with prescription ED drugs. In order to avoid a potentially risky drop in blood pressure that could theoretically lead to fainting, stroke, heart attack, or even death, prescription nitrate medications such as the ones listed below should not be combined with prescription ED drugs (These medications have many brand names and come in many forms.):

• Nitroglycerin
• Isosorbide mononitrate
• Isosorbide dinitrate
• Erythrityl tetranitrate
• Pentaerythritol tetranitrate
• Sodium nitroprusside
• Amyl nitrite (inhaled, poppers)
• Any other medication with organic nitrates

Nitrates that are found in or added to vegetables, meat products, and other foods are not a concern. The amount of nitrates in food is too small to make a difference when combined with ED drugs. Nitrates are added to some foods to improve flavor, color, and shelf life, and to protect against bacterial growth. Unless you eat so much meat that your cholesterol is 1000 mg/dl, it is okay to eat a piece of meat without having to worry about having a stroke.

FACT #6: It makes the most sense to start with the lowest doses of these drugs.

Starting out with low doses is generally recommended for any over-the-counter or prescription medication. I always like to say that with any pill you should "start low, go slow, and you will save a lot of dough." You should always be put on the lowest dose of ED drugs if you are older, have liver or kidney issues, or are on drugs that could inhibit or impact other drugs and how they are metabolized (erythromycin, ketoconazole, itraconazole … check with your pharmacist and doctor). It is also very important to remember not to take more than 1 dose a day! Prescription penis pills can be helpful but have serious side effects if you take too much.

Men who have liver or kidney failure and men who are on medication that inhibits the primary drug metabolic pathway in the body should be given the lowest doses of these drugs. It is very important to always tell your doctor what pills you are taking before beginning any ED drug. Other medications that you might be taking could interact dangerously with ED drugs or nullify their effectiveness.

How long do prescription penis pills take to work, and what is the duration of effectiveness?
- Cialis: Onset is 30 to 60 minutes. The highest blood concentration is reached in about 120 minutes, and the efficacy is good for 12 to 36 hours.
- Levitra: Onset is 30 to 120 minutes. The highest blood concentration is reached in about 60 minutes, and the efficacy is good for about 5 hours. (Also available as a dissolving tablet under the name Staxyn.)
- Viagra: Onset is 30 to 120 minutes. The highest blood concentration is reached in about 60 minutes, and the efficacy is good for about 5 hours.

Are ED drugs effective? Absolutely!

What is the catch? There are 2 big catches!
Catch #1: Cost
ED pills cost only $10 to $25 per pill (sarcasm intended). In my opinion, the embarrassingly high cost of these pills is not, nor has it even been, justified. Even though the ridiculous pricing structure has lasted as long as it has, the high cost of ED drugs never gets enough attention, especially from some of the physicians who speak so highly of these drugs to other physicians. Very few companies that manufacture lifesaving (cholesterol, blood pressure, etc.) or non-lifesaving medications would ever get away with charging this amount of money for a single pill. I believe the cost of these pills is one of the reasons why 33 to 50 percent of individuals do not refill their prescription after they fill it the first time.

Initially Viagra was supposed to be a drug for chest pain. Even though it did not prove to be efficacious for its original purpose, Viagra was not trashed because men in the original studies began to get better erections. The rest is history! Viagra's chance origin negates justifying the price of the pills based on research and development costs. Why do they charge such an extremely high price for each pill? Is it possible they would have made more money by charging less for this pill because it would have increased the likelihood that some men would continue to take it long-term? I will let you answer that question!

Catch #2: Short-Term and Potentially Long-Term Side Effects

The lack of an effect and high cost are the most common reasons for quitting ED drugs. However, approximately 25 percent of men stop taking these pills because of side effects. The side effects from ED drugs are largely similar and include:

• Headache (the most common problem, occurring in about 10 percent of men)
• Flushing (more common with Viagra)
• Nasal congestion (more common with Viagra)
• Dizziness (fainting is rare)
• Gastrointestinal upset (more common with Cialis and Levitra)
• Back pain (more common with Cialis)
• Muscle pain (more common with Cialis and Levitra)
• Altered vision (less than 2 percent of men, occurs mostly with Levitra and Viagra)
• Hearing and vision loss are a rare side effect for all ED drugs.
• Seizures are a very rare side effect.
• Non-arteritic anterior ischemic optic neuropathy (NAION) is a rare condition that has been reported after the use of all prescription ED pills and may result in decreased vision or permanent vision loss.

Is it true that when they were compared in head-to-head (no pun intended … I think) studies, sugar pills fared well against Viagra?
Yes, this is true. On average, 25 percent of men on the placebo sugar pill had a similar response to those on prescription ED drugs. This finding indicates that the mind can really influence the body. More research on ED is needed to determine what really works better than a sugar pill.

Why do ED drugs not work at all in some individuals?

Incorrect usage is one of the two primary reasons why these drugs fail. ED drugs are used incorrectly if there is insufficient sexual stimulation, the dosage is not high enough, or not enough time has passed between taking the drug and attempting sexual activity. The second main reason why ED drugs fail is that they simply don't work for some people.

Experts recommend a minimum of 6 attempts with a specific drug dosage before it is officially considered a failure because results generally get better with ongoing use. An increase in dosage should always be considered if the current dose fails. If you hang in there and don't quit these pills before completely exhausting all your options, you might still be one of the couples that benefit from these great drugs.

ED drugs do not work as well in men with ED caused by:
- The removal or injury during prostate surgery of nerves that help with erections
- Diabetes with neuropathy
- Peripheral vascular disease
- Worsening cardiovascular problems
- A sensitivity to side effects
- Low testosterone

New research suggests that men who go on testosterone replacement therapy (TRT) or increase their level of testosterone and also take an ED drug may significantly improve their erectile function. Since every pill and drug supplement comes with a catch, make sure you read Chapter 9 to learn much more information on TRT.

Does food or alcohol impact the metabolism or efficacy of these drugs?
Perhaps.

- Cialis: When consumed in moderation, food and alcohol do not impact this drug.
- Levitra: High-fat meals can reduce the maximum concentration of this drug from 18 to 50 percent, and alcohol may impact its efficacy.
- Viagra: High-fat meals reduce or prolong the absorption of this drug, and alcohol may impact its efficacy.

Talk to your doctor or pharmacist about the latest on drug interactions.

You may not qualify for ED drugs if you currently have or have had any of the following conditions or are taking certain medications for them:

- Nitrates administered in any form (IV, oral, gel, etc.) to treat chest pain
- Low, high, or uncontrolled blood pressure
- Cardiac failure
- Unstable chest pain
- Retinitis pigmentosa
- Cardiovascular disease, heart attack, stroke, or arrhythmia

Can ED drugs be combined with prostate enlargement drugs?

There is a class of prostate enlargement drugs that help men urinate better known as alpha-blockers (alfuzosin, doxazosin, silodosin, tamsulosin, terazosin, etc.). When used with ED prescription pills, alpha-blockers could produce a drop in blood pressure. This drop occurs upon standing and could lead to fainting and other negative side effects. To optimize safety, men generally should not take any ED drug within 4 hours of taking an alpha-blocker. Some experts have offered the following more specific recommendations:

- Doxazosin and Terazosin are older alpha-blockers that can have a greater impact on lowering blood pressure than the more prostate-selective alpha-blockers alfuzosin, silodosin, and tamsulosin. If there is a concern about combining alpha-blockers and ED drugs, alfuzosin, silodosin, and tamsulosin are preferred because they are safer options. Talk to your doctor for advice on the best option for you.
- You must be on a stable dose of alpha-blocker prostate medication before you can use any ED drugs. Only after determining that you have been on that medication long enough with minimal side effects should your doctor begin seriously discussing ED drug options with you.

What should I do if I am following all the instructions and these ED drugs still aren't working?

- Talk to a specialist who is willing to listen to you.
- Make lifestyle choices that are healthy for your heart and overall well-being more often. Exercising more, eating healthier, and reducing the amount of stress in your life are all great healthy lifestyle choices.
- Try using ED drugs and a quality-controlled supplement together.
- Get your testosterone and other health markers checked.
- Change to another prescription ED drug.
- Use the drug regularly for masturbatory purposes even if you do not expect sexual activity.
- See a sex counselor.

Is it true that these drugs may help with many nonsexual conditions and may even help some women and children with other medical issues?

Yes! Since these drugs help to dilate some blood vessels to improve blood flow and to deliver oxygen to some tissues, they have been used to treat other health conditions that could benefit from this mechanism of action. Here are just some of the conditions that these drugs may help:

Altitude sickness

It should not be a surprise that ED drugs can potentially help with altitude sickness, for they improve blood flow and oxygen delivery to some tissues, including the lungs. I am curious ... if someone climbs Mount Everest on Viagra, does that officially still count as having climbed the mountain or will his or her name have an asterisk next to it like a major league baseball player who breaks a record while on steroids? What is the difference between Sir Edmund Hillary using Tenzing Norgay to help fuel his drive to climb Mount Everest and me accomplishing the same amazing mountain climbing feat or even just making it up the steep street nearby where I live in Ann Arbor, Michigan, while on Viagra? (These are the sorts of things I often contemplate when my mind wanders in abnormal directions! Now you know why I was never smart enough to get into Harvard Medical School.)

Dying flowers

Based on some small past studies, a solution of Viagra (only 1 to 2 percent of that found in the pill) appears to improve oxygenation to wilting flowers. Because these drugs are so expensive, it makes a lot more cents (pun intended) to save your money and just buy new flowers. However, if you are anything like me, you might pass on buying new flowers and try to capture this rebirth on camera to sell it to some entertainment news channel for millions of dollars.

Jet lag

Some laboratory research suggests that these drugs speed up the time it takes the body to become accustomed to jet lag. Nevertheless, there have not been any notable clinical trials to support these preclinical findings. In order to avoid making your airline blanket do some embarrassing tricks witnessed by others on the plane, I suggest sticking with 1 mg of melatonin instead.

Memory issues/Alzheimer's

Because these drugs improve blood flow to certain parts of the body and brain, it might be possible for them to improve memory and reduce the risk of Alzheimer's disease. I would love to see more research in this area because increased sexual activity and masturbation would probably do the same thing. In other words, I would rather have sex with my wife than take these pills for memory enhancement. Besides, a desire to improve your memory is one of the last perfect excuses that you can use in your marriage.

Prostate problems (enlargement)

As men age, a condition that can impact urinary flow called benign prostatic hyperplasia (BPH), or noncancerous enlargement of the prostate, becomes almost as prevalent as the common cold. It seems that some men can improve their flow if they take these drugs when other drugs are not working well enough. The greatest benefits have been observed in men who have both ED and BPH issues.

Pulmonary arterial hypertension (PAH)

There is a drug that is approved for this condition to help improve the ability to exercise; people suffering from this condition can be short of breath, dizzy, and can tire easily. This drug works by relaxing the blood vessels in the lungs and allowing more blood to flow to these areas to get more oxygen there. Young and older adults have used the drug Revatio. However, Revatio is actually sildenafil, which is also known as Viagra! Wow! I am going to stay politically correct and not comment on the fact that some young adults taking Revatio for PAH may be getting a surprise every once in a while.

Raynaud's disease

This is a condition that results in abnormal blood flow, especially to colder extremities such as the fingers and toes. Some men and women with Raynaud's Disease seem to benefit from taking ED drugs because they increase the size of and relax blood vessels, and improve blood flow.

How about that fairly popular prescription pill found in Europe called Apomorphine that dissolves under the tongue?

I am happy that I remembered to discuss this pill before wrapping up this chapter. Some folks pick up this medication while traveling in Europe, bringing new meaning to the saying "when in Rome!" I personally think Apomorphine, also known as Uprima in some countries, should have been approved in the United States. However, I will bring up (pun intended) the side effects of this drug, which form part of the reason it did not get approved in the U.S.

About 20 minutes before sexual activity, Apomorphine pills are placed below the tongue. This centrally acting drug gets into the blood stream quickly and affects the brain and spinal cord. While most prescription ED drugs work outside of the brain and spinal cord to produce an erection, Apomorphine acts on the sacral parasympathetic nervous system. Unlike the other peripherally acting prescription penis pills, Apomorphine is a nonselective Dopamine agonist (D-2) that binds to receptors in the hypothalamic region of the brain and enhances naturally occurring pro-erectile signaling mechanisms.

Since Apomorphine works in the brain, it cannot be combined with numerous other drugs that work in the brain. Antidepressants and other psychiatric medications should not be taken at the same time as Apomorphine, and alcohol and other fatigue-inducing drugs make the side effects much worse. Taking more than one pill within a 24-hour time period can also greatly worsen the side effects.

Erections occur within 20 minutes of taking this medication in more than two-thirds of individuals. Apomorphine has a faster onset of drug activity but a lower rate of effectiveness and satisfaction than ED drugs offered for sale in the United States. Apomorphine is most effective in men with mild-to-moderate ED.

Apomorphine can be taken by some men who do not qualify for prescription ED drugs approved in the United States because they take nitrate medication or for other reasons. Even with the approval of a doctor, taking Apomorphine and nitrate medication at the same time is controversial.

Unwelcome side effects that get worse with higher doses, such as nausea (17 percent of individuals), vomiting (6 percent), headaches, dizziness, and sweating are a primary reason why compliance with Apomorphine is an issue. This drug was not given FDA approval because during testing in the United States it caused a lot of problems at a dose of 6 mg.

I have to admit, if I experienced nausea and vomiting when taking ED drugs they would probably kill the romance! Sometimes it's hard to see the difference between side effects from Apomorphine and similar medications in the United States because ED drugs have been so expensive in this country that they make me want to vomit. Despite its side effects, I think it's seriously a shame that Apomorphine is not available in the United States because it could have helped many couples who do not like or could not use other options.

As you can see, there is a lot to consider with prescription ED pills. However, there are also plenty of other options for men with ED problems. Many of the other options do not receive as much attention as the penis pills, but offer the right option for some individuals. In the next several chapters, we'll give an overview of those other choices.

CHAPTER 5

Vacuum Erection Devices

This is a case where the name really sounds worse than it is. We'll spend a few pages giving you some information on this option and you can decide for yourself.

How do vacuum erection devices (VEDs) work?

A VED, sometimes called a vacuum constriction device (VCD), consists of 4 parts:
1. The open end of a clear, tube-like cylinder is slipped over the entire non-erect penis.

2. To help blood enter the penis to get hard, a vacuum pump is attached directly to the cylinder to remove air from inside it.

3. To create a tight seal between the cylinder and the skin at the base of the penis, gel is placed on the circular lip of the open end of the cylinder before it is slipped over the non-erect penis. Applying a gel at the open end of the cylinder should also make it easier to get a good erection. You can avoid having pubic hair painfully pulled by the cylinder if you trim nearby pubic hair beforehand. Trimming pubic hair can also help to prevent a disruption in the seal.

A manual or battery-operated vacuum pump uses negative pressure to pull blood into the penis from the arteries and veins of the body by removing air from inside the cylinder. Because the manual pump requires two hands, one to stabilize the cylinder on the penis and the other to pump the device, most experts favor the one-handed battery-operated option.

4. An appropriately sized constriction band or tension ring is placed on the open end of the cylinder so it can be slipped around the base of the penis once an erection occurs to help maintain hardness. A band or ring that is too small will be painful, and one that is too large will make it difficult to remain sufficiently hard. The band should be placed as close as comfortably possible to the base of the penis because the penis should be hard beyond the area of the constriction band and soft behind it.

As was mentioned, to help create the tightest comfortable seal between the device and the base of the penis, it is important to trim pubic hair in this area before the pump is activated. If the band is placed too far away from the base of the penis, it will cause an unstable soft area to form that could bend and make penetration difficult. Since only minimal oxygen reaches the penis when its blood flow is restricted, the band should be removed within 30 minutes to avoid damaging the penis.

More useful information on VED

What do I need to know in order to buy the right VED?
With a prescription from your doctor, you can pick up a VED from your local pharmacy or order it directly from one of its FDA-approved manufacturers. To avoid risking the health of your penis, do not use a VED or any of its accompanying parts if you did not acquire them with a prescription. You could damage your penis by using items from a non-prescribed VED kit, such as metal or inelastic bands and not the recommended flexible bands.

What if my partner or I want to extend our sexual activity beyond the medically recommended 30-minute limit?
Wow and wow spelled backwards! Although this is actually a fairly common question, I personally get sleepy just thinking about it. If you desire to continue sexual activity past the safe 30-minute cutoff, it is possible to repeat the procedure after waiting several minutes or more. Remember, you risk damaging your penis by leaving the band on any longer than 30 minutes. Another option is to forgo using the constriction band entirely. Thanks to penile rehabilitation following cancer surgery, injury, or other medication conditions, some men may be able to improve their erections without always using the band.

How long does it take to get an erection using a VED, and will it be a hard erection?
On average, it takes 2 to 3 minutes to achieve an erection using a VED. While most men can get erect faster than boiling an egg, individual results vary. Some men may take as long as 10 minutes or more. It should be kept in mind that experts suggest it takes 4 or 5 attempts to learn how to use this device before one can become comfortable and capable operating it. Some research shows intermittent pumping improves the hardness of the penis. You may actually get a better erection during sex and/or masturbation by using the pump for 1 to 2 minutes, releasing pressure, and then pumping again for 3 to 4 minutes.

What are the hard advantages?
• VED is effective when used by men with ED, regardless of the cause.
• This is a non-invasive method of treating ED.

- The side effects of using this device are minimal.
- There is good insurance coverage for the VED.
- In general, there aren't any restrictions on how often it can be used.
- Battery-operated and push-button versions of this device are now available for anyone with severe arthritis of the hand.
- Even though most experts prefer using prescription pills and occasional injections for penile rehabilitation, the VED could be added to most rehabilitation programs.
- If something more is needed to improve erections, a VED can be combined with pills, pellets, injections, and some surgeries that are already being used to treat ED. Many individuals who took an ED pill 1 to 2 hours before using a VED reported having better erections, and were more likely to regain natural erections at a later time.

What is the soft catch?
- Because vacuum pumps cause primarily non-oxygenated venous blood to enter the penis, your erection might be slightly colder to the touch or when inserted, and it might be more a more bluish color than the more typical reddish cast of an unassisted erection. The constriction band may further add to this effect.
- Long-term satisfaction rates with the VED are fair, ranging between 50 to 66 percent.
- The VED usually requires good manual dexterity.
- The creation of the vacuum or use of the device may cause penile pain.
- Numbness may be experienced during an erection.
- The penis is not as consistently hard along its entire shaft because less blood enters some of the penile tissues than in a natural erection. However, the penis may be wider than it would normally be.
- The constriction band can cause delayed ejaculation, interference in ejaculation, or pain during ejaculation.
- There is often a decrease in the intensity of orgasms.
- Bruising may occur.
- In some more rare cases, achieving an erection can take as long as 10 to 20 minutes.
- There may be a loss of an acute angle of erection.
- In order to insert the penis for intercourse, a hand may also be needed for stability.
- A non-physiological erection where there is a large amount of superficial vein swelling may occur.
- Pubic hair and/or scrotal skin can get pulled into the vacuum cylinder and cause pain.
- Traveling with the bulky equipment, bands, and gel required for the VED to function is not easy or very private.
- Versions of the VED that have not been medically tested or approved and are

constructed without safety valves can be ordered in catalogs, on the Internet, and in some erotic equipment stores. Safety valves are important to have in these devices because they prevent excessive pressure from causing penile injury. Speak with your doctor to ensure that you always purchase a reputable FDA-approved VED that has a safety valve.

- The track record for these devices is actually not bad. After 2 years, 50 to 66 percent of men continue to use them. Compared to older men, younger men appear less likely to use them long-term.

Individuals with the following conditions are usually not good candidates for a VED:

- Men with bleeding disorders and those on blood thinners should not use a VED because bruising or swelling from trauma to the veins may occur. If you are only taking aspirin and are not on two or more blood thinners, your doctor may be comfortable prescribing a VED.
- Men should not use a VED if they have a history of priapism, a disorder resulting in a prolonged erection, or blood disorders that lead to prolonged erections, such as sickle cell disease, thalassemia, or leukemia.
- Men with too many red blood cells or any other blood cell disorder should not use this device.
- If you have a significant amount of penis curvature, use of the straight cylinder device could exert stress on your penis. Men with Peyronie's disease who have undergone surgery and been through successful conventional treatment should talk to their doctor about the potential to benefit from a VED.
- To avoid penile injury, men with reduced penile sensation due to a spinal cord injury or other medical conditions shouldn't use a VED. In these cases, trauma caused by long-term use of the constriction band may be difficult to feel until something such as skin ulcerations occurs.

Fast Fact: VEDs have been used in one form or another for over 100 years! (Is that not longer than we have been using vacuum cleaners?) Is it a surprise that everything seems to originate from sex?

CHAPTER 6

Prescription Penis Pellets

Yes, really, this is not a joke. Either you or your partner can insert this semisolid pellet into the tip of your penis after you urinate. Once inserted into the urethra, the Medicated Urethral Suppository for Erection (MUSE, for short, or Prostaglandin E1 or transurethral alprostadil) can give some men good erections quickly because 80 percent of it is dissolved and absorbed within 10 minutes. MUSE works by relaxing smooth muscle tissue and increasing the size of blood vessels to allow more blood flow. It is important to remember that each MUSE applicator in each foil pouch is to be used only one time. The erection should begin within 5 to 10 minutes after the pellet (only 3 or 6 mm long, 1.4 mm in diameter) is inserted into the penis from an applicator stem (slightly longer than 1 inch, 3.5 mm in diameter), and can last from 30 to 60 minutes.

Directions for using MUSE

1) Before inserting the pellet, try to urinate. Then you should gently shake your penis several times to ensure there is only a small amount of excess urine. A urethra that is slightly wet after urination will allow MUSE to work better, as this medicine was designed to dissolve faster in the little bit of urine that remains.

2) Open the one-time-use-only foil pouch and remove the MUSE applicator. Keep the foil pouch nearby so that it can be used for discarding the MUSE applicator. With your thumb and forefinger, remove the body of the applicator from the cover where the medicine is located. Look at the transparent applicator to make sure you can now see the pellet at the end of the stem.

3) Now that you have prepared the applicator, it is time to insert the pellet into the penis. In a sitting or a standing position, slowly and gently stretch the penis in an upward/northward direction to its full length. Then softly squeeze the head of the penis from the top and bottom so that the urethra opens at the tip of the penis. Slowly insert MUSE into the urethra and then push down the button at the top of the applicator so the pellet is released into the urethra. To ensure the pellet is inside the penis, gently swivel the applicator from side to side for about 5 seconds. Remove the empty applicator while the penis is still upright.

4) Hold the penis upright, stretch it to its full length again, and roll the penis between your hands for at least 10 seconds. This will ensure that the medication gets effectively distributed inside the penis. If you feel a burning sensation, it may help to roll the penis for another 30 to 60 seconds, or until the burning goes away.

5) Following the insertion of MUSE, it is recommended that you walk around for 5 to 10 minutes. This is meant to increase blood flow and to further distribute the drug inside the penis.

6) Remember, the MUSE package is good only for a one-time use. Make sure you replace the cover on the applicator, put it into the now-open foil pouch, fold to close, and then discard it into your normal waste container.

More useful information on MUSE:

- Frequency: A maximum of 2 separate packets can be used every 24 hours.
- The average time it takes to start getting hard is about 7 minutes.
- The maximum time to penile engorgement is about 20 to 23 minutes.
- Erections can last longer at the higher dosages.
- If MUSE is not successful, the chances of improving your results increases by using a constricting band like the ACTIS adjustable constriction loop around the base of the penis to prevent venous blood from leaving the penis.

What are the hard advantages?
- Although the success rate is lower than with penile injection therapy, about 70 percent of individuals are satisfied or very satisfied when treated with MUSE.
- Even men who have had their nerves damaged or removed from prostate surgery may experience a response from MUSE.
- MUSE works in 5 to 10 minutes and can last from 30 to 60 minutes.

What is the soft catch?
- Cost: MUSE is not cheap. Each pellet costs as much as a fine-dining restaurant meal.
- Between 30 and 40 percent of men experience aching, pain, or discomfort in the penis, testicles, legs, or the area between the penis and the rectum.
- You may experience a warming or burning feeling in the urethra.
- The penis may become red from increased blood flow. (Is that such a bad thing?)
- Urethral bleeding or spotting occurs in around 5 percent of men due to improper use.
- Some of the 5 to 6 percent of women who experience vaginal burning or itching from the drug transferring to vaginal tissues might benefit from water-based vaginal lubricant.
- Less common side effects include a prolonged erection, dizziness, light-headed

ness, fainting, a rapid pulse, and a reduction in blood pressure.
- Avoid using MUSE if your partner is pregnant (unless you use condoms), if your penis is abnormally shaped, or if you have a blood disorder such as sickle cell anemia or trait, low blood platelets, or too many red blood cells.

Please consult your doctor if you have any questions related to MUSE.

CHAPTER 7

Penile Injection Therapy

Okay, I can feel you cringing at just the mention of penile injection therapy. Truthfully, it sounds scarier than it is. Bear with me and we'll get the facts out there.

Penile injection therapy is one of the most effective therapies for men with very serious erectile issues or those who need penile rehabilitation to treat nerve damage to the genital area. The injection goes into the base of the penis or penile cavernosal tissue near the body. It relaxes the smooth muscle and increases blood flow to the penis. After completely understanding all of the risks of priapism, you and your partner could eventually complete this injection at home. Priapism is an erection that is not caused by sexual arousal, will not go down, and could damage penile tissue.

Yes, these injections work well, but don't forget this is serious medicine. No book or booklet should claim that the information it provides replaces the need for a few visits to your doctor. In this chapter, we will cover just the important basics of penile injection therapy.

How often can I give myself this injection?

Usually you can give yourself an injection a maximum of 3 times a week, with at least 24 hours between usages.

What drugs are used in the injections?

- The most common drug is Alprostadil (PGE1, brand names Caverject and Edex). This drug works by opening up the blood vessels and bringing blood into the penis. If someone has erectile dysfunction that requires more medical help, several other drugs can be added to the injection.
- Papaverine (Pavabid), a drug derived from the poppy plant, is another drug that can be used to open up or expand blood vessels to allow blood to enter the penis.
- Phentolamine (such as the brand Invicorp) is another drug used to open up or expand blood vessels to let blood enter the penis. This drug is also used to bring down blood pressure in cocaine-induced and other hypertensive emergencies.

Can a man simultaneously receive more than one of these drugs to help with erections?

Yes! The medical lingo is as follows:

Unimix
- Alprostadil (Caverject Impulse)
- An erection occurs within 5 to 20 minutes of an injection and can last up to 2 to 3 hours after an ejaculation.

Bimix
- Papaverine and Phentolamine

Trimix
- Alprostadil, Papaverine, and Phentolamine
- This three-drug combination can increase efficacy up to 90 percent. If papaverine is used, fibrosis of a part of the penis is 5 to 10 percent more common.
- Also available as a gel, which can be applied to the tip of the penis to promote an erection in individuals who have either failed on prescription ED pills or cannot tolerate the pills due to side effects.

Quadmix
- Alprostadil, Papaverine, Phentolamine, and Atropine
- Atropine is a drug that is only rarely needed.
- This 4-drug combination is rarely used because there is an increase in side effects, and the extra benefits compared to risks are not impressive in many cases (there are exceptions, of course).

What is the most effective and well-researched drug(s)?
Combination therapy, especially Trimix, has both the highest efficacy rate and the highest risk for priapism and fibrosis. You should work with your doctor to decide whether or not you need this treatment, and, if you do, what drug combination is most appropriate for you.

Do these injections improve sex drive?
No. Think of these injections as supercharged Viagra. Although the injections can really help the male equipment of many men work better, they will not make a man want to use his equipment any more than he already does. Despite lacking a sex-drive stimulating component, these drugs have helped many couples when no other treatment has worked for them. This wonderful result alone might be

enough to make men want more sexual activity, even if they still need serious help with erections. These injections are one of the most effective methods to achieve penile rehabilitation for some men with nerve injuries from accidents, diseases, or prostate cancer treatments.

Why is there such a concern about taking too much of these drugs or having a prolonged erection?

Health-care professionals and individuals work together to determine the lowest effective injectable dose to prevent prolonged erections and other unwelcome side effects. A prolonged erection (usually lasting more than 4 hours) is a medical emergency that should be treated by a doctor to avoid permanent damage to the penis. In some cases, a needle can be used to remove blood and reduce pressure in the penile tissue and cause the penis to soften. If the penis becomes rigid again, doctors can inject phenylephrine or a similar drug to cause it to go soft.

Can these injections be combined with pills, pumps, pellets, etc.?

Most doctors allow some combination of treatments for men who really need to benefit from a flexible approach. The specific products that can and cannot be included in a combination treatment plan must be discussed with a doctor. For instance, because one of the drugs used for injection therapy is identical to the penis pellet drug, simultaneously using these treatments could produce very bad consequences. Injections are so effective that they are usually taken alone or combined only with lifestyle and dietary changes. It is more common for men to occasionally rotate injection therapy with other products, such as a pill or pump, than it is for them to combine multiple products at the same time. I believe the possibility of staying interested in penile rehabilitation and remaining active opens up by rotating between different treatment options.

What are the hard advantages?

- It has one of the highest initial satisfaction rates for couples that qualify for it!
- These injections work for men with ED from all sorts of causes, including men who have had their erectile nerves damaged or removed during prostate surgery.
- An erection can occur with OR without sexual stimulation.
- An erection can last up to an hour.
- A return of spontaneous erections can occur in some men.
- Erections that arise with the help of these injections are similar to naturally occurring erections. In both cases, blood comes in through arteries and is prevented from leaving through veins.

What is the soft catch?
- You (or your partner) have to administer the injections into the corpora cavernosa of the penis.
- Prolonged erections that risk damaging penile tissue occur in 5 percent of men.
- Priapism occurs in 1 percent of men.
- Penile pain and painful erections may occur.
- Fibrosis that can be problematic occurs in the penile area of 2 percent of men.
- Bruising and injection-site bleeding may occur.
- Superficial infections may occur near the injection site.
- Tolerance to the drug can develop.
- Urethral bleeding can develop.
- Some men may experience a drop in blood pressure.
- Dizziness may be present.
- There is a low long-term compliance rate of 40 to 68 percent.

Individuals with the following conditions are usually not good candidates for penile injection therapy:
- Those who have priapism and other conditions associated with an increased risk of long-term unhealthy erections
- Individuals with sickle cell anemia
- Leukemia patients
- Men with penile implants
- Men taking MAO inhibitors and some other prescription drugs
- Non-compliant candidates, such as alcohol and drug abusers
- Individuals with a fear of needles. Although many diabetics start out fearing needles, they gradually become accustomed to them after first learning how to inject other objects such as apples, oranges, bananas, etc. If a fear of needles is holding you back from trying these injections, talk to your doctor about how you might overcome your fear.

CHAPTER 8

Penile Implant Surgery

Also called penile prosthesis surgery, penile implant surgery should receive serious consideration only by men with erectile dysfunction who have failed with or rejected all the more conservative options—pills, vacuum erection devices, pellets, and injection treatments. For anyone seriously considering penile implants, it is essential to discuss the advantages and disadvantages of this option with a qualified specialist. If a man qualifies for this procedure, he should work very carefully with a doctor to select the specific penile implant that meets his needs.

A Comparison of the Types of Penile Implants Available

Non-Hydraulic
This type of implant utilizes semi-rigid, malleable, or bendable rods. Men who lack manual dexterity due to a physical condition may like these "grab and point" implants. Non-hydraulic implants provide flexibility and durability because they are made with silver and stainless steel wires, silicone, polyethylene, and alloy cables. The penis is always basically erect with this type of implant, especially when it is pointed in a straight direction or bent upwards. If both you and your penis can adjust to having a constant erection, then this might be the implant for you! This is the least expensive option.

Hydraulic
The three basic pieces that make up this type of implant are the reservoir, pump, and cylinders. To cause an erection to occur, fluid is squeezed from the reservoir into the cylinders. When you are done, press the release button and the fluid will go back to the reservoir. Two basic types of hydraulic implants are commonly used.

- Multi-component, 2-piece, inflatable hydraulic implants: These devices are composed of a single scrotal pump bulb and paired hollow cylinders. They are similar to the 3-piece type in the manner in which they go into the penis. To achieve an erection, this implant needs to be pumped up. The pump is small, located in the testicular area, and sometimes it isn't easy to inflate. The fluid in the cylinders can be transferred back into the reservoir by gently bending the penis downwards for 10-15 seconds. Because all parts of this device are implanted in the body, this option offers the benefit of being well concealed.

- Multi-component, 3-piece, inflatable hydraulic implants: These devices are composed of paired hollow cylinders that are placed in the penis, a scrotal pump and valve, and a reservoir that is surgically placed in the lower abdomen. The scrotal pump brings fluid in, and the valve releases fluid back out. Afterward, the release valve in the scrotum is gently squeezed to release fluid back into the reservoir located in the lower abdomen and the penis becomes soft again. Most individuals prefer 3-piece inflatable devices because they feel more natural when the penis is and is not erect. This implant is well concealed because all parts of the device are implanted in the body. Satisfaction with this device is about 90 percent or more, and the device durability at 10 years is 75 percent. This is a more expensive option.

Which implant makes the most sense for what type of man?

The 3-piece inflatable penile implants are generally recommended for younger men with normal manual abilities, men who wear form-fitting clothing, and men who shower in public. Inflatable penile implants are recommended for anyone with advanced Peyronie's disease or neurological diseases, and men considering secondary implants. Malleable implants may be better for obese individuals, men who do not have good manual control, and those for whom the cost of inflatable devices is too extreme.

What do the experts say about the hydraulic device surgery?

- Individuals usually shower with antibacterial soap for a few days before the surgery.
- The genital area is shaved immediately prior to the surgery to reduce the chance of a bacterial infection.
- Antibiotics are usually given 1 hour before the surgery.
- Semi-rigid rod implants can occasionally be put in with local anesthesia but hydraulic implants should use general or regional anesthesia (short-acting spinal anesthesia is preferred by many experts).
- Many individuals are instructed to wear brief-type underwear for about 30 days following the surgery. They are also encouraged to try to point their penis upward for proper care.
- Individuals are taught how to use the hydraulic devices about 4 to 6 weeks after surgery.
- Most individuals do not have any pain or discomfort by the third month post-surgery. If pain persists past this point, it could indicate the presence of an infection or nerve issues that may occur with individuals who have diabetes or other conditions that increase their risk of encountering these problems.

What else do the experts say about penile implants?

- An auto-inflation, or a partial spontaneous inflation that occurs without your control, is a rare side effect of the 3-piece inflatable penile implant. Talk to your doctor about this.
- The head of the penis does not get as full as it would during a normal erection because the device is implanted in the shaft and not the end of the penis. In some cases, the head can even droop slightly. This droop can sometimes be fixed with a re-implantation of longer cylinders. Men who are uncomfortable with a less firm head and men who feel a cooler temperature on their penis after this surgery may benefit from using an erectile dysfunction drug or MUSE.
- Erections with the device may be shorter than your previous naturally occurring erections.
- Many studies have shown that both men and their partners have a high rate of satisfaction with the penile implant. Couples report the ability to get erect quickly and the capacity to achieve good hardness as two common reasons why they are satisfied with the implant.
- Lower levels of satisfaction have been expressed when there is a reduction in overall penile length. This unwelcome reduction in length is especially likely to occur when there needs to be a surgical redo following an infection, when Peyronie's disease is present, and as a result of other factors. It is best to discuss this with a specialist.
- Although the reasons are not known, some studies have shown that obese individuals have a higher dissatisfaction rate with penile implants. Some experts suggest fat pad size may cause some mechanical issues in some obese men. Before men who are obese undergo the implant operation, perhaps they should discuss waist/weight loss with their doctors.

Are there other surgeries?

There are other penile surgeries that can restore some blood flow to the penis and improve erections. These other options are too complicated to be presented in a book, but instead ought to be discussed with a specialist. If you are interested in any penile surgery, make sure you seek expert advice, especially if you have any concerns or complicating conditions.

What are the hard advantages?

- Penile implant satisfaction rates are very high, ranging from 70 to 90 percent.
- This is a good option for men who have not liked other treatments or have simply run out of other options.

- Men with penile deformities can get implants.
- Venous-leak syndrome can be helped with this operation. Venous-leak syndrome makes it very difficult to naturally get erect and stay firm because penile venous blood leaks out of the penis and back into the blood vessels of the body.
- Men with severe erectile dysfunction can benefit from a penile implant. For example, men who have undergone pelvic surgery or who have severe diabetes, Peyronie's disease, fibrosis, or priapism can benefit when nothing else seems to work.

What is the soft catch?

- The penile implant surgery has some irreversible effects. Due to scarring associated with the device, other treatments are rarely helpful if the prosthesis is removed.
- Men can still have orgasms and ejaculate, but the ability to have natural erections is lost.
- Penile implant surgery is the most invasive of all options. In some cases, hospitalization is needed.
- About 9 percent of men need repeat surgery.
- After 5 years, mechanical failure is less than 5 percent with 3-piece prostheses and 1 to 10 percent overall.
- Erosion of the corporal/urethral tissue area occurs in 1 to 11 percent of penile implants.
- Although the risk of infection is present, antibiotic prevention strategies limit the infection rate to only 2 to 3 percent. Infections can be further reduced to 1 percent or even less by using an antibiotic or hydrophilic-coated implant.
- An infection can require removing the prosthesis, using antibiotics, and re-implanting it after 6 to 12 months. There is also a high success rate managing infections with a method called salvage therapy. This method involves removing the prosthesis, irrigating certain areas of the penis with a multi-antibiotic solution, and immediately re-implanting the prosthesis.
- Although diabetes is supposed to be a serious risk factor for infections, so far this has not been demonstrated with penile implants.
- The average lifespan of the device is usually 7 to 10 years and perhaps longer in healthy men.

CHAPTER 9

Testosterone and Testosterone Replacement Therapy

As we start talking about low testosterone and its impact on male sexual health, we should start with just a few general facts.

- Testosterone is a hormone produced largely in a man's testicles. Testosterone levels in men increase before and during puberty, and then decrease gradually after about the age of 40 by 1 to 2 percent each year.

- Over the course of a man's life, testosterone plays an important role performing all sorts of essential functions that you may or may not be aware of. At puberty, boys have an increase in testosterone that helps to deepen voices, initiate erections spontaneously, and increase muscle mass, sex drive, exercise capacity, and the number of oxygen-carrying red blood cells in the body by 15 to 20 percent. (In fact, mild anemia that can become common in elderly men is probably due to lower testosterone levels.)

- A man's blood testosterone levels are customarily not measured unless a problem is suspected. If a decision to test is made, there are several tests that may be chosen by your doctor to measure your testosterone level and help to determine a possible cause for the deficiency. Men normally experience their highest level of testosterone sometime between 6 and 10 AM, so testosterone testing is generally done before 9 AM.

- Low testosterone in men can be caused by several factors including genetics, obesity, lack of sleep, and aging. Whatever the specific cause may be, the result is a disruption in normal brain signaling that helps to stimulate testosterone production and/or a reduction in the production of testosterone. Low testosterone can occur at many ages.

What is "andropause" and what are its symptoms?
After they receive a hormonal message from the brain during puberty to begin operating, certain cells in the testicles become the primary producers of testosterone. If these cells are not able to make enough testosterone, men can experience andropause. There are many potential reasons why men have low testosterone. Understanding these potential reasons is valuable because testosterone is just as important for men as estrogen is for women.

Some of the potential symptoms of low testosterone levels are listed below:

• Reduced libido
• Erectile dysfunction
• Difficulty reaching orgasm
• Reduced intensity of orgasm
• Reduced sexual penile sensation
• Reduced energy, sense of vitality, or sense of well-being
• Increased fatigue
• Depressed mood
• Impaired cognition
• Diminished muscle mass and strength
• Decreased bone density
• Anemia

Based on the diversity of potential low testosterone symptoms, a questionnaire called Androgen Deficiency in the Aging Male (ADAM) was developed years ago. If the questionnaire suggests you have low testosterone, there is a good chance that you do. However, if the questionnaire does not suggest you have low testosterone, you might still have it. The major issue I have with this questionnaire is that it sets up too many men to believe that the answer to all of their problems is testosterone replacement therapy. So although you can still use it, keep in mind that this questionnaire has limitations.

ADAM QUESTIONNAIRE:

1. Do you or have you had a decrease in sex drive?
2. Do you or have you had a lack of energy?
3. Do you have a decrease in strength or endurance?
4. Have you lost height?
5. Have you noticed a decrease in your enjoyment of life?
6. Are you sad and/or grumpy?
7. Are your erections less strong?
8. Have you noticed a recent deterioration in your ability to play sports?
9. Are you falling asleep after dinner?
10. Has there been a recent deterioration in your work performance?

If you answered yes to question 1 or 7, or any other 3 questions, you may have low testosterone. However, you can also see how your answers may vary depending on the day. I would have answered yes to question 1 and 7 on Monday after a 10-mile run, but not on Tuesday when I was rested and made love to my wife! This week I would have answered yes to questions 3, 6, and 9 because I have been working late and not getting any sleep writing this book.

Do you think that ADAM used questions that are intended to convince you that you need more testosterone? I believe that this questionnaire should be used more as an informative tool to bring attention to the problem of low testosterone and should not make or break your decision to seek testosterone treatment.

What should you know about the blood test for andropause?

It is difficult to determine if a man has andropause without a testosterone blood test that is drawn before 9 AM. In order for your doctor to determine how much testosterone you are capable of producing on your own, he or she will try to draw blood when testosterone levels are highest, in the morning. Later in the day testosterone levels can be reduced significantly.

What are some options if low testosterone is a problem?

In my opinion, the best way to increase testosterone is to lose weight and increase muscle mass. Talk with your doctor about the options.

Prescription testosterone replacement therapy is usually the best approach to medically increase severely low testosterone levels in men who have already tried to increase their testosterone by losing weight or waist. In some men, TRT may accomplish one or more of the following: increase muscle mass, reduce belly fat, and improve mood, energy levels, and sexual enhancement. There isn't another prescription medication that can increase men's testosterone levels as safely and effectively as TRT.

However, on top of not being cheap, TRT is overprescribed as a cure-all for multiple problems that some men could correct by making lifestyle changes. No type of testosterone replacement product is approved for the treatment of erectile dysfunction. Individuals on certain prescription medications, with a history of breast or prostate cancer; an enlarged prostate; urinary, liver or kidney problems; sleep apnea; and some other medical conditions are not necessarily good candidates for TRT. Blood tests will occasionally be needed to monitor testosterone levels, cholesterol, red blood cell levels, and liver function. TRT is not a good option if you and your partner are trying to have a baby because it can reduce scrotum size and inhibit mature sperm development. (However, TRT is unreliable as a method of male birth control.)

What lifestyle changes can increase my testosterone?

Losing weight and/or waist can have the biggest impact on increasing testosterone levels. While other lifestyle changes such as quitting smoking, getting adequate sleep, and lowering stress levels can have a small impact, effective dieting can increase total testosterone levels as much as 100 points or more!

What dietary supplements can increase my testosterone?

Large quantities (hundreds of mg daily) of a fairly cheap dietary supplement called DHEA can increase low testosterone levels. However, not only is it a pain to take a lot of pills, DHEA can also increase liver toxicity and estrogen levels in men. I have watched many men with low testosterone slightly bump up their testosterone by taking DHEA, but it has always made me nervous because it appeared to have little symptomatic benefit and a lot of risk at the higher doses that were needed to produce the slight increase in testosterone.

The other available herbal medicines and supplements that mimic DHEA are no more exciting, and you will end up paying more money for the same sort of product. Examples of products with DHEA-resembling compounds in them are those that are yam-based or contain the herb Tribulus terrestis. I personally think that these products might be beneficial only in rare cases when men have low DHEA levels or for women who have some sort of sexual dysfunction. It appears that at 25 mg per day, DHEA might do something slight for a small number of women with female sexual dysfunction (FSD). This topic is beyond the scope of this text, so discuss DHEA further with your physician if it is of interest to you.

What different types of currently available prescription medications can increase my testosterone?

Many different forms of testosterone replacement therapy will be covered in the following pages

Buccal (testosterone transbuccal or transmucosal system)
- This medication can most closely mimic the actual rise and fall of daily body testosterone levels.
- The mouth can become irritated where the product is applied along the upper gum. Striant is an example of this medication.
- This treatment option is very expensive.

Gel (transdermal topical)
- This medication should be applied to specific areas of the body when skin is clean and dry. Follow specific product directions to determine application areas; the recommended area varies by product.
- The gel needs to dry completely before dressing.
- To prevent the gel from being transferred to anyone else, you need to wash your

hands thoroughly after each use with soap and water. In my opinion, it is best to follow the wash with an alcohol-based hand sanitizer.
- Women and children should not be exposed to the gel.
- Occasionally, minor skin irritation is experienced with these gels.
- AndroGel comes in 2.5 g and 5 g packets and a pump that has 60 1.25 g pumps.
- Testim comes in 50 mg packets.
- Fortesta and Axiron are relatively new testosterone gels on the market and may be worth considering.
- Androgel can go on the shoulders, upper arms, or abdomen, and Testim can go on the shoulders or upper arms, but not on the abdomen. Check with your doctor for specific application instructions.
- This is an expensive option.

Intramuscular Injection
- Testosterone enanthate and cypionate (injectable esters) are used.
- With this option, testosterone is injected into the muscle.
- These injections tend to be lower in cost than other testosterone therapies.
- Frequent medical visits may be needed to administer injections that are required on an average of every 1 to 4 weeks. Because it is easy to reach maximum blood testosterone levels, a roller coaster effect may occur when blood testosterone levels peak in the first 5 days after an injection.
- Mood swings, breast tenderness, and breast enlargement may be associated with the peak of blood testosterone levels that occurs in the first few days after an injection.
- The injection site can be painful.
- Of all the testosterone replacements that are available, this option comes with one of the highest risks of side effects.

Oral (Pills)
- Due to the increased risk of liver toxicity caused by oral testosterone, these products usually aren't prescribed and generally shouldn't be used.
- Oral testosterone products can also increase the risk of stomach upset and irritation.

Scrotal Skin Patch
- Medication is delivered through a patch placed on the skin of the scrotum.
- This option is easy to use, and it delivers regular testosterone levels over time.
- Although it is rare, skin irritation, itching, and discomfort may occur.
- Inadequate absorption of the medication through the skin may occur.
- Androderm and Testoderm are two examples of this medication.
- This is a less expensive option.

Non-Scrotal Patch

- This patch is not placed on the scrotum, but is discreetly positioned on upper-body skin.
- This option is easy to use, and it delivers regular testosterone levels over time.
- Although it is rare, skin irritation, itching, and discomfort can occur.
- Inadequate absorption of the medication through the skin could occur.
- If irritation with the patch occurs, please ask your doctor about a preventive cream such as 0.1% triamcinolone acetonide that can be applied to the skin prior to the patch.
- A daily application is needed.
- This is a less expensive option.

Pellets

- In order for the medication to be delivered, several pellets are placed just under the skin in the hip area or upper buttocks slightly below the beltline. The pellets need to be removed after they are used.
- An example of this medication is Testospel.
- This method delivers testosterone for 3 to 6 months.
- Although this procedure only takes about 10 minutes and no stitches are needed, the doctor does have to numb the area with a local anesthetic.
- This option is expensive.

What are the common and not-so-common catches involved with using testosterone replacement therapy (TRT)?

Potential Risks and Side Effects	Comments
Acne or oily skin	Rare or infrequent
A non-cancerous enlargement of the prostate known as benign prostatic hyperplasia (BPH)	Rare
Breast pain, breast enlargement (gynecomastia), and a slight risk of breast cancer	Usually the pain or enlargement is reversible when dosage is lowered or discontinued, but breast cancer in men is serious and requires treatment.
Cardiovascular disease	Evidence actually suggests TRT has no negative impact on cardiovascular health, and may potentially have a beneficial effect, especially in younger men. In older men with many other medical problems, there is some concern that TRT could be slightly harmful to the heart (this is controversial).
Cardiovascular disease	Most studies show no positive cholesterol changes result from taking TRT, and there is a slight chance of a reduction in good cholesterol (HDL). Men who lose weight or waist on testosterone may experience favorable cholesterol changes.
Estrogen levels may increase in men due to the conversion of some testosterone into estrogen.	This side effect may actually cause breast problems in some men.
Edema from fluid retention	This is rarely a problem except in individuals with conditions that put them at a high risk. Some high risk conditions include heart failure, kidney problems, and other medications, such as ACTH, that carry a risk of edema.

Liver toxicity	This side effect occurs more often from oral pill-based testosterone, but is rarely still a problem because this form of testosterone is no longer used in many countries.
Prostate cancer	Controversial, unknown, and requires regular monitoring (PSA, DRE, etc.) regardless of the type of TRT used.
Erythrocytosis and polycythemia	These two conditions can occur when red blood cells are abnormally increased. Requires monitoring and tends to be higher when taken in injection form.
Sleep apnea	This neurological condition occurs infrequently due to anatomical changes in the upper airway that can be fixed with the proper device. Individuals with obesity and lung disease and those who use the injection form of TRT are at higher risk.
Skin irritation or reactions	The risk of skin side effects is higher with a patch, low with a gel, and rare with injections or pellets.
Sperm count reduction	TRT can cause temporary infertility.
Testicle atrophy, leading to a reduction in testicle size	This is a common side effect, especially in young men, but can usually be reversed when treatment stops. Infertility may occur.
Natural testosterone can be reduced or no longer produced by the body, even when discontinuing TRT.	Ouch! Talk to your doctor about this side effect because it seems that many men are not aware of this risk. This is why many experts favor a 3-month trial period on TRT to see if it even is working for a man before risking any long-term side effects.

What are some tests used to monitor individuals on TRT?

Initial Tests:
- To execute the initial TRT tests, visit a urologist or endocrinologist who works with TRT.
- A urinary history and understanding of baseline urinary issues will be determined.
- Questionnaires will be used to gather information.
- A history of sleep apnea will be determined.
- A CBC blood test, digital rectal exam, PSA test, and testosterone blood level test will be done. Some experts also suggest doing cholesterol testing.
- Other blood tests may be needed.
- An ultrasound and MRI may be performed.

Follow-Up Tests:
- For the first year, you should follow up with your doctor every 3 to 6 months. Your doctor and you will determine the frequency of your visits after the first year.
- Tests that are similar to the ones performed initially should be repeated during follow up visits.

OTHER FREQUENTLY ASKED QUESTIONS ABOUT TRT

Can TRT accelerate or encourage male pattern baldness?

It is absolutely possible and makes complete sense that TRT can accelerate or encourage male pattern baldness in men with a genetic risk of this condition, but this has not yet been adequately studied. Even though genetics, and not testosterone replacement, is the primary cause of this baldness, testosterone is needed to express the gene for baldness in a number of hair follicles. It's true that the chances you will go bald will be considerably reduced if your testicles, the site of most of the body's testosterone production, are removed. However, at this point, I am not ready to recommend testicular removal as a cure for baldness!

Should I have a prostate biopsy before I start TRT?

Doctors generally won't require a prostate biopsy prior to starting TRT. However, physicians will require some men who are at high risk or have already been treated for prostate cancer to have a biopsy to be sure TRT is given safely. Individuals who require a biopsy are the exception, and not the rule.

Can I go on TRT after prostate cancer treatment?

The answer to this question is controversial. Generally, the answer is no. Usually doctors are of the opinion that men should not use TRT if they are known or suspected to have or have had prostate cancer. On occasion however, some doctors may permit individuals with very low testosterone levels following treatment for a prostate cancer that was not aggressive to take TRT while under their close supervision. Doctors generally don't recommend TRT to individuals who have undergone prostate cancer treatment unless a few years have passed since the last treatment, and their very low testosterone levels are clearly negatively impacting their quality of life. However, these cases are the exceptions, and should always be worked out with a doctor you trust.

Can salivary testing be used to measure low testosterone?

Most of the studies that are used to determine low testosterone are based on blood tests and not spitting!

Which questionnaires are helpful in determining if I have low testosterone?

In addition to the ADAM questionnaire discussed earlier, two online questionnaires that can be used to help diagnose the condition are the Aging Male Survey (AMS) and the Massachusetts Male Aging Study (MMAS). A completed questionnaire from an individual may add another piece to the puzzle. Doctors, especially specialists, may find it helpful to receive completed questionnaires because they often contain clues that help them to connect information and solve problems.

How can testosterone increase the risk of breast cancer?

In some rare cases, especially in heavy men, an enzyme called aromatase converts excessive amounts of testosterone to estrogen. This conversion can stimulate breast tissue in men and eventually contribute to the development of breast cancer. Testosterone replacement therapy must always carry the warning that testosterone can be converted into estrogen. Men who use the prescribed amount of medication and maintain a healthy lifestyle should not be concerned, for the chances of this happening are very small. Men who are known or suspected to have breast cancer should not use TRT.

What should people know about taking TRT and having a baby?

Because TRT causes many men to become infertile, the longer a man is on the medication, the more difficult it will be for him to have a baby. In order to avoid this problem, do not go on TRT if you want to have a baby. Women who are pregnant, may become pregnant, or are breast-feeding should not use TRT or be exposed to TRT products.

What if I qualify for TRT, but I do not want to take testosterone itself to raise my blood levels. Is there any other prescription drug I can take?

Remember, TRT can reduce male fertility and can permanently shut down the body's natural ability to make testosterone in some men. There are two non-testosterone-based products that a small number of men should be offered by doctors. Some young men, men concerned about permanent testicle shrinkage, or men concerned with maintaining their fertility have the option of taking the oral drug clomiphene citrate (also called "Clomid" or "Serophene"). This pill is better known for improving female fertility than male fertility. However, in some men, it may stimulate the production of a hormone in the brain (luteinizing hormone or LH) that travels to the testicles to stimulate testosterone production. Men with low to normal LH levels are usually the ones who benefit, but men with high LH levels as measured by a blood test usually do not benefit from this drug. This pill has a low rate of side effects, but experts comment that slight weight gain or blurred vision might occur. Another option, but one that is arguably more difficult and not used as often, is injections of intramuscular (buttocks or shoulder) human chorionic gonadotropin (HCG). This is another drug more commonly given to women to improve fertility or ovulation. This drug is similar to the hormone LH mentioned, so it can increase testosterone in some men who have normal or low LH levels. However, like clomiphene, it is not a good option for men with high blood levels of LH. Some experts recommend getting these injections 3 times a week and checking to see if it is working after one month. An alternative perhaps for certain individuals only.

CHAPTER 10

Premature Ejaculation, Peyronie's Disease, and Other Male Sexual Issues

PREMATURE EJACULATION (PE)

Fast Facts: With about 20 to 30 percent of men having PE at some point in their lives, it is arguably the number-one male sexual dysfunction. Unlike erectile dysfunction, PE is not affected by age. Unfortunately, most men with PE never seek help, a fact we need to change.

What is PE?

This condition isn't as simple to define as it seems because what constitutes PE can be subjective. A commonly accepted definition of PE is an ejaculation the sufferer has little or no control over, occurring earlier than desired with minimal stimulation, before or soon after penetration, and causing bother or distress. The International Society for Sexual Medicine provides a slightly different definition: "a male sexual dysfunction characterized by ejaculation which always or nearly always occurs prior to or within about one minute of vaginal penetration; an inability to delay ejaculation on all or nearly all vaginal penetrations; and negative personal consequences, such as distress, bother, frustration and/or the avoidance of sexual intimacy." Common to these definitions of PE is the emphasis on the time it takes to ejaculate, the lack of an ability to control or delay an ejaculation, and the presence of negative impacts such as bother and distress.

Some experts believe that there are 2 types of PE—primary and secondary—that differ based on whether they are lifelong or acquired. Primary PE first occurs during men's earliest sexual experiences and continues to be a problem all throughout their lives. Ejaculations that occur too soon, either before vaginal penetration or less than a minute or two afterwards, are typical with PE that is lifelong. Secondary PE can be either suddenly or gradually acquired, with an onset that marks a change from previously normal ejaculations. Although the ejaculations occur too soon with acquired PE, they usually aren't as premature as the ejaculations that occur in lifelong PE.

Why does PE happen?

Researchers do not know what causes PE. There is little data to support previous theories that claim PE is caused by anxiety, penis hypersensitivity, or a neurochemical imbalance. Recently, acupuncture has shown a benefit in treating PE, although the exact mechanism is unknown.

How is a diagnosis of PE made?

In order to diagnose PE, a specialist will review your medical and sexual history and perform a physical exam. There are a variety of questionnaires that your doctor may choose from to help make the diagnosis and determine the course of treatment. Your doctor will consider how long it takes you to ejaculate, how much sexual stimulation is present, the impact on quality of life, and anything that you consume or do that might influence PE. Before settling on a diagnosis of PE, it is critical for your doctor to ensure you have PE and not ED. A specialist will probably use the information he/she gathers to determine if you have lifelong or acquired PE and if it is nonspecifically present or occurs under specific circumstances and/or with a certain partner(s). Prostate inflammation, ED, or any other condition that is diagnosed along with PE, should be addressed separately, which may help with the treatment of PE.

What is the treatment for PE?

There are several fairly simple and potentially beneficial inexpensive behavioral techniques that you can discuss with your doctor.

One option, the stop-start technique, involves taking breaks from sexual activity after starting. This technique may involve a partner stimulating the other's penis until he is about to reach orgasm and then stopping at this signal. Starting and stopping stimulation to delay orgasms can be repeated over and over with time delays built in. This technique has gradually helped some men overcome their tendency to ejaculate prematurely.

Another option that helps to delay ejaculation is the squeeze technique. Although this technique has several versions, the primary method of deterring ejaculation involves using your thumb and forefinger to squeeze the head of the penis when the sensation of ejaculation first begins. By focusing pressure on the urethra, this technique temporarily reduces sexual tensions and the ejaculatory response by pushing blood out of the penis.

Some young men use the technique of intentionally reaching an orgasm during masturbation prior to intercourse in order to make it less likely that they will ejaculate too quickly when they have sex with their partner. Some men are told to practice delaying ejaculation for up to 15 to 20 minutes during masturbation. By tapping the benefits of masturbation, when game day comes, you can perform on the field as well as you do in practice! (Sorry for the cheesy athletic analogy.)

It is in the best interest of you and your partner to remember that the most sensitive vaginal nerve endings are in the lower third of the vagina. Instead of thrusting vigorously and ejaculating prematurely, penetrate the first 2 to 3 inches of the vagina with slower, shallow movements. Not only is this technique likely to please your partner, it could help you last longer.

Other behavioral tips include tightening the pubococcygeal (PC) muscles of the pelvic floor with the Kegel exercises that were discussed in the first chapter. Both men and women can locate these muscles by practicing stopping the flow of urine. Once you learn this exercise, you can practice Kegels in your car, walking, at your desk, and anywhere else you wish, even when you don't need to urinate. Practicing Kegels in sets of 10 will increase the strength of your PC muscles and give you better ejaculatory control.

Another common behavioral technique that can be used to treat PE is called sensate focusing. This option involves both partners setting aside time every week in order to learn to patiently explore, touch, and kiss a variety of each other's body parts without any pressure. Not having the pressing need for intercourse or orgasm may help to slowly make each partner comfortable with the other's body. The sexual process can be further desensitized if the partners masturbate in front of one another. Massage oils and lubricants are encouraged. Some couples eventually move from sensate focusing to the squeeze technique.

All of these behavioral techniques help a man and his partner realize where his "point of no return" is and how he can develop better control over it. Behavioral techniques intended to deter premature ejaculation aren't always successful long-term. In order to maximize success, they can be combined with other treatments. To learn more about this, talk with your doctor or visit a reputable Internet site.

Prescription Treatment Options for PE
Prescription drug treatment is one of the first options for men with lifelong PE. Even though most of these treatments are not specifically approved for PE, many doctors and individuals have had success with certain off-label medications. Only certain Selective Serotonin Reuptake Inhibitors (SSRIs) and on-demand topical anesthetics have consistently shown a benefit for the treatment of PE. (SSRIs are a class of compounds more commonly used as antidepressants.) Daily prescription medications are usually the first choice for many specialists treating PE. Some of the more common drugs used are:

- Fluoxetine
- Paroxetine
- Sertraline

The anti-depressant Paroxetine appeared to work better than many other drugs. Why might a doctor prescribe antidepressants to treat PE? Even though this class of drugs is better known for working as antidepressants, they are also used to treat other conditions because they affect several different areas of the body. These medications have been prescribed to treat hot flashes, PE, and multiple other conditions that aren't usually associated with depression. If you truly need treatment for PE, don't let the drug name, the condition it is commonly known to treat, or its somewhat narrow reputation stop you from using the SSRIs your doctor prescribes.

Keep in mind that a delay in the time to ejaculation may start a few days after beginning these drugs, but is more common after a week or two. The side effects of these drugs are usually mild, improve after a few weeks, and may include the following:
- Fatigue
- Drowsiness
- Yawning
- Nausea
- Vomiting
- Dry mouth
- Diarrhea
- Perspiration

Rare but reported side effects include a reduced sexual drive, reduced chance of orgasm and ejaculation, and erectile dysfunction. While some men prefer to take these drugs as needed or on demand, daily dosing tends to work better. It makes the most sense to use the lowest possible doses of these medications when treating PE.

Dapoxetine, sometimes called Priligy, can be taken on demand and does not need to be taken daily, unless you have sex every day. This drug is arguably the most powerful SSRI that has been more specifically used to treat PE. Both of these doses have been effective for some individuals from the very first dose. The most common side effects are:
- Nausea
- Dizziness
- Diarrhea
- Headache

Fewer than 10 percent of individuals in clinical trials quit taking Dapoxetine because of side effects. Dapoxetine has been approved in the following European countries: Austria, Finland, Germany, Italy, Portugal, Spain, and Sweden. It is also apparently approved for use in New Zealand, but still has not been approved in the United States.

Topical Anesthetic Desensitization Creams for PE

There are a variety of desensitizing creams, such as 5 percent lidocaine-prilocaine cream, that can stay on the penis for 20 to 30 minutes during intercourse to reduce the sensation that could lead to a fast ejaculation. However, if they are left on for 30 to 45 minutes, a loss or difficulty in maintaining an erection due to penile numbness could result from the cream being on too long. It is best to use a condom to prevent your penis from transferring the anesthetic agent to your partner, causing her/him to experience some temporary numbness.

Talk to your doctor about the results of research that is testing different formulations of lidocaine and prilocaine for information on whether an aerosol or other product is available in this area.

Some ginseng-based herbal supplement creams that with contain other ingredients could work by reducing penile sensitivity to stimulation. Note that any anesthetic, a small percentage of individuals experience some localized burning or pain. Make sure to discuss with your doctor recent research on products to better understand their risks and rewards.

What about erectile dysfunction drugs for PE?

ED drugs have not had an overwhelming impact on reducing the time to ejaculation in studies thus far. They did seem to improve confidence, the perception of ejaculatory control, and overall sexual satisfaction, and they reduce anxiety and the amount of time needed to get a second erection. Other studies show conflicting results and some have observed better results when combining ED drugs with a SSRI or another treatment. The bottom line is to talk to your doctor about the latest research on these drugs.

PEYRONIE'S DISEASE (PD)

PD is a deformity of the penis that some studies suggest can impact as few as 1 percent to as many as almost 10 percent of men. It is most common for this disease to occur in men ages 55 to 60, but it has also been reported in men who are younger and older than this age group. PD is caused by fibrous lesions that form along the penis. Individuals with this disease generally have 3 primary complaints:

- Painful erections that are not necessarily severe but are bothersome
- Plaques on the penis that can be felt and may be soft, tender, calcified, very hard, etc.
- Penis curvature, with the direction depending on plaque location and number

Men select from among the multiple treatments that are available based on how they are affected by these 3 primary complaints. When a diagnosis of PD is made, penile curvature is found in about 80 percent of men, and painful erections are reported by about 50 percent

Curvature of the penis is caused by fibrous penile plaques that pull on penile tissue on the same side affected by the plaques. These plaques are located on the top/ dorsal surface of the penis 66 percent of the time. Lateral (side) or ventral (bottom) plaques are less common but result in more sexual issues because the curve or angle changes make sex more difficult. Multiple plaques may be present.

PD presents itself in either an acute inflammatory phase or a chronic phase. The acute phase is characterized by penile pain and curvature and by the formation of a nodule. This more suddenly occurring phase involves waxing and waning periods of symptoms that can resolve over 6 to 18 months. Interestingly, in the chronic phase, there is little to no pain, nodule size stays roughly the same, and there is some degree of penile deformity.

Why PD and all of its accompanying symptoms occur in some individuals? It is common for experts in this area to think that the "trauma theory" might explain the occurrence of PD. According to this theory, an injury site develops when a partially or fully erect penis regularly experiences repeated trauma or microtrauma during intercourse. Although it is difficult to determine who falls into this category, trauma theorists say that some individuals are genetically at a higher risk of having PD. This injury process leads to microscopic tears and bleeding below the skin, and eventually causes a clot to form that sets off a large immune response to clean up the damage. Plaque formation results when a large amount of collagen is laid down to repair the damage at a specific injury site. Some experts believe that this process of damage and repair makes Peyronie's Disease a wound-healing disorder.

Doctors can reduce the curve or problem by using penile injection therapy or a vacuum erection device. In order to help confirm the diagnosis and guide treatment, doctors may ask individuals to bring in pictures of their penis problems that they took at home. Stress associated with PD is sufficiently high that it is not uncommon for men to experience depression with this condition. In addition to the deformity being a problem, research suggests that the penile shortening that comes along with it can also be very difficult for men to deal with.

Peyronie's disease is associated with diabetes in 30 percent of individuals and erectile dysfunction in 50 percent of individuals! PD is also associated with high blood pressure, high cholesterol, obesity, smoking, pelvic surgery, and low testosterone levels. The most important take-home message is that urologists can really help you with PD today!

Fairly Exciting Non-Surgical Treatments of Peyronie's Disease

Note: These treatments make more sense for men in the early stages of the disease, while the plaque is still forming. Since many studies using these treatments were not of a high quality, they come with some controversy. Some studies discuss options for pain improvement, but PD pain can decrease over time without treatment. Some studies discuss reducing penile plaque size, but this reduction does not correlate with improvement in the curvature of the penis. Many urologic experts recommend referring to studies that show a reduction in penile narrowing, shortening, curve, or other specific deformities as the best method for judging treatments. Over time, about 50 percent of men with PD get worse without treatment and 50 percent do not. It is important to have a specialist follow you to ensure you make the right decisions, because the best way to manage PD isn't always clear.

Acetyl Esters of Carnitine Dietary Supplements
Some studies suggest penile plaque size, curvature, and pain can be reduced by the dietary supplement L-carnitine (2g), specifically propionyl-l-carnitine, and the drug verapamil.

Colchicine
Past studies have shown a benefit with the drug colchicine, but recent studies show that results are similar to those of a placebo when it is given by itself. In combination with vitamin E supplements, colchicine may reduce penile plaque size, curvature, and pain during the initial phase of the disease. Discuss the latest information on vitamin E supplements with your doctor because they are currently receiving attention for potentially increasing the risk of other health problems.

CoQ10 Dietary Supplements
New research suggests that some men with early chronic PD can benefit by taking CoQ10 supplements at a dosage of 300 mg per day. This fairly large study found that, compared to a placebo, after 24 weeks CoQ10 significantly reduced penile plaque size and curvature and improved erectile function. Wow! Who knows if this study was too good to be true? Even if it was, this supplement has such a good overall safety record that it is certainly worth a try. Perhaps CoQ10 should be used instead of vitamin E whenever a doctor wants to add a supplement to conventional therapy. Using vitamin E as a cream instead of a pill is the one exception to the suggestion

of using CoQ10 instead of vitamin E because it is a safer way to use the supplement. I suggest comparing prices of CoQ10 supplements, because these supplements are not cheap. CoQ10 piils and vitamin E cream could potentially be used together.

Collagenase, Interferon, or Verapamil Injections

An injection of the drug collagenase may have the ability to decrease plaque size and penile curvature by breaking up collagen. Verapamil, an injection that is commonly used today, may reduce penile curvature as well. Injections of the drug interferon alpha-2b may also be beneficial, but this option is more expensive than using verapamil.

Pentoxifylline or Other Prescription ED Drugs

More research is needed to see whether Pentoxifylline, Viagra, and other ED drugs could prevent PD from getting worse by acting somewhat similarly to increase nitric oxide (NO) levels. Even though this interesting theory isn't proven, some men with PD also have ED, so why not try to see if any of these drugs could be helpful? I wonder whether some of the NO-increasing dietary supplements mentioned in the third chapter could help. This has not been adequately tested at this time.

Potassium Para-Aminobenzoate (Potaba)

My dad, an 80-year-old practicing urologist who still loves his job, once wore a T-shirt that said something like "Keep straight with Potaba." Since Google was not around back then, I didn't know what that saying meant. Now that I do know the meaning of that shirt, I wonder where it is today. Although no one is sure how it works, according to one theory, Potaba decreases fibroblast cell collagen synthesis. Recent research shows that although it may reduce plaque size, it doesn't reduce penis pain or curvature. Taking 3 grams of Potaba daily for a year has been one of the more effective doses.

Other Miscellaneous Treatments

The ESWL device used to break up kidney stones is being studied to reduce pain in PD. When used with some conventional treatments, a topical energy source called iontophoresis applied to the genital region during a doctor's visit may improve pain.

Not-So-Exciting Non-Surgical Treatments of Peyronie's Disease

Steroid injections

These have not shown to have a benefit for PD.

Tamoxifen

Although this drug is customarily used to treat breast cancer, a study from the early 1990s suggested that 20 mg taken twice daily could help reduce penis pain, curvature, and plaque size in the early stages of PD. Recent results have not been as promising, and this drug has lots of potential side effects.

Traction Therapy Devices
This device slowly expands a specific penile tissue area, but research on this technique is ongoing.

Vitamin E Supplements
Recommending 400 or 800 IU of vitamin E, with or without conventional therapies, arguably used to be the most common non-surgical treatment of PD. Recent research suggests the positive results may just be the result of a placebo effect. The latest research on high doses of vitamin E supplements shows that they may actually be unhealthy for your heart and prostate and may even cause internal bleeding. In my opinion, most men should look at the forest rather than the tree and stay away from these supplements! However, if you do still want to use vitamin E, it is a lot safer when applied as a cream daily to the site of concern.

Surgical Treatment of Peyronie's Disease
Surgery is the gold standard for fixing the PD penis deformity. Only men who have had their disease stabilized for about 6 months should consider this procedure. Surgery is also better for men with hardness issues, men who have a painless deformity, men who cannot engage in sexual activity regularly or at all due to the deformity, and when non-surgical options will not correct this problem as a result of a calcified or hardened plaque.

What is the Surgical Catch?
Although surgery can reduce penis curvature enough for many men to resume sexual activity, it doesn't always fully correct the problem. Surgery can sometimes cause a slight reduction in penile length and hardness, and in rare cases, it may reduce some penile sensation. You should talk to your doctor to determine whether surgery is a sensible option for you and which surgery would be the most suitable for your situation.

You should also discuss in detail with your doctor the importance of carefully following a postoperative care program and penile rehabilitation after surgery. Some of the various postoperative care and rehabilitation options that could possibly be used include getting your partner involved in reducing the stress and anxiety of restarting sex, taking ED drugs, and using a pulling device to prevent penile shortening. These options should be discussed in depth with a qualified surgeon.

OTHER MALE SEXUAL ISSUES

Prostate Problems (BPH, Cancer, Prostatitis/Pelvic Pain)

Whenever you have prostate issues, such as a non-cancerous enlargement known as benign prostatic hyperplasia (BPH) that can impact urinary flow, it is not unusual to see an impact on sexual or erectile function. Therefore, preventing or treating prostate conditions is really important. If you have been or will be treated for prostate cancer, you must talk to your doctor about penile rehabilitation. In my opinion, this can completely change your sex life. Today everyone knows that physical rehabilitation can improve your life if you are injured in any way from an accident or athletic event. Despite this, for some reason, penile rehabilitation still does not get the credit it deserves even though mild to serious ED and other penile issues can improve in men following surgery, radiation, hormone therapy, and most other prostate cancer treatments.

My book *Promoting Wellness for Prostate Cancer Patients* discusses many options for rehabilitation that can improve penile issues. In addition, it provides a great deal of other valuable information on how to improve prostate health, sexual health, and overall well-being. Another great resource on penile rehabilitation, *Saving Your Sexual Life: A Guide for Men With Prostate Cancer,* was written by one of the world's best experts in this area, John P. Mulhall, MD. This doctor and his book are awesome! I'd suggest you check it out.

Prostatitis is an inflammation of the prostate gland that can be very painful. Acute prostatitis, chronic prostatitis (CP), and chronic pelvic pain syndrome (CPPS) are problems in men that should be taken seriously. Acute prostatitis can increase a man's PSA blood test count and increase his anxiety because he thinks he might have cancer, when really it is just an infection. Physicians are very good at treating acute or infectious prostatitis, but are challenged by CP and CPPS. CP/CPPS can be hard to diagnose and can cause pain in the pelvic region, testicles, penis and even the area between the anus and testicles (perineum). Your sexual and urinary health may be impacted, and the pain can be severe enough to impact your overall quality of life. There are experts today (generally urologists) who specialize in these areas, and there are all kinds of potential treatments used. The treatments range from prescription medications (muscle relaxants, prostate medications, pain relievers, etc.) to dietary supplements (Q-Urol, for example; see www.farrlabs.com) to stress reduction and exercises that have evidence of efficacy. Nothing equals an expert in CP or CPPS who can first determine if you have either condition, and then recommend the right treatment approach to resolve the problem.

Infertility

Even though I recommend seeing an expert on these issues, I want to add something very important on this topic. Recently one of the largest reviews of dietary supplements and male infertility found that using some supplements could significantly improve the chances that men could impregnate their partners. Along with assisted reproduction techniques (ART), these supplements can help couples have a baby. Wow and wow spelled backwards! While this is a groundbreaking finding, the problem with this review is it did not suggest which supplement, of the numerous that have shown a benefit, men should take to improve their infertility. In my opinion, this isn't a tough decision if you stick to looking at the forest rather than the trees. Any supplements that have not been shown to be healthy for your heart and overall health should not be recommended or taken to treat male infertility.

I recently wrote a chapter in a medical urology book to help you make the best decisions for your health when selecting supplements for male infertility. Of the supplements mentioned in this large expert review, my article suggested taking 200 to 300 mg of CoQ10 per day, 2000 to 3000 mg of L-carnitine per day, 1000 to 2000 mg of fish oil per day, or 500 to 1000 mg of vitamin C per day because they all have been found to be healthy for your heart and safe overall. Talk to your doctor about taking one or several of these supplements while trying to have a baby. Folic acid, selenium, and vitamin E are supplements that were also mentioned in this review but NOT RECOMMENDED in my article because they do not have a heart-healthy history and, in some studies, have been found to be unhealthy for your prostate. Thanks to this new information, it is now much easier for men to understand how to combine healthy dietary supplements with some assisted reproductive techniques. Following a heart-and-sex healthy diet and lifestyle plan can also help. Regardless of how helpful they may be, none of these recommendations will ever replace seeking advice from a specialist if you need it.

Sexually transmitted disease (STDs)

Do you really need me to say something here, folks? Men and women need to be careful by practicing safe sex techniques and/or finding a monogamous partner. I should not need to tell you why or how STDs could impact your sexual function and life expectancy. It takes 10 years of rigorous medical training after college to be able to deliver someone else's baby or treat a serious disease, and only a few seconds of not thinking to conceive a baby or contract a serious disease. Enough said!

Counseling or Sex Therapy?

"Hey, Dr. Moyad, why did you bury this topic at the end of the chapter and toward the back of the book?"

Although I didn't do this on purpose, the goal of this book was to discuss options that I can really help you with ASAP. Although I am not a sex therapist, I completely believe that counseling and sex therapy could make or break your sex life or relationship. However, finding a counselor or therapist who is just right for you is not easy. But fabulous professionals like Dr. Lori Buckley of Pasadena, California, are out there! Ask your primary care doctor for help, and take enough time to investigate who may be the right fit for you and your partner. Make sure you understand that a counselor or therapist is like a marriage partner. When the fit feels right, the relationship can be helpful, and when it does not fit, it can go terribly wrong. Never forget that mental health is linked with sexual health, and vice versa. Depression, stress, anxiety, and anything else that contributes to poor or inadequate mental health can have a negative impact on your sex life, and a poor or inadequate sex life can negatively influence your mental health.

CHAPTER 11

Female Sexual Dysfunction

It is a fact that we hear a great deal more about erectile dysfunction than about female sexual dysfunction. Perhaps that is because advertising for expensive ED drugs is so common on evening television. However, studies show that only 20 to 30 percent of women reach orgasm regularly with a partner. About 30 to 50 percent of women report sexual complaints, but the number of women who actually seek medical treatment is much lower. We do know that at least 30 percent of women have some issues with sexual desire, arousal, or orgasm. In some studies, low libido was the most common complaint reported, and low arousal was the second-most common complaint.

Many experts and some professional medical organizations believe that unless women experience personal distress from their sexual problems or dysfunctions, they shouldn't view them as an issue that needs be treated. As many women age, they are often satisfied and happy regardless of having some sexual problems or dysfunctions that might have caused them more distress sometime in the past.

It is safe to say that female sexual dysfunction (FSD) is a common problem, with estimates of women who have some form of FSD ranging from about 25 to 63 percent. Sexual issues that could be classified as an FSD usually fall into one, and sometimes multiple, of the following 4 FSD subtypes:

1. Libido
2. Arousal
3. Orgasm
4. Pain

When evaluating FSD, lubrication and overall sexual satisfaction are two other areas that are considered. In fact, some sources consider these areas to be FSD subtypes, while others do not include them on the list. Either way, they are always considerations in the total picture.

Once again, some studies show low libido to be the most common complaint and low arousal to be the runner-up. It is not uncommon for women to have problems with orgasms, pain, or overall sexual satisfaction, nor is it uncommon for a combination of FSD subtypes to be experienced by the same person. FSD can occur regularly, periodically, or situationally. It may be caused by physical and/or psychological factors, or arise from unknown causes.

Sexual desire disorders are divided into 2 categories:
• Hypoactive sexual desire disorder (HSDD) is the lack of desire for sexual activity and/or the lack of sexual thoughts or fantasies.
• Sexual aversion disorder is the fear and avoidance of sexual thoughts, situations, and/or contact.

Sexual arousal disorder is the persistent or recurrent inability to achieve or maintain sexual excitement. A reduction in genital lubrication and/or swelling may be present.

Orgasm disorder is the difficulty or lack of an ability to achieve orgasm after sufficient sexual stimulation and arousal. A primary orgasm disorder is when an orgasm has never been achieved despite sufficient effort. A secondary orgasm disorder is when an orgasm has been achieved at some point in the past, but a difficulty or inability to reach orgasm has developed sometime since that point. An absolute orgasm disorder is when an orgasm can't be reached in any situation. Situational orgasm disorder is when an orgasm can only be achieved in certain situations.

Pain disorders are divided into 3 categories:
• Dyspareunia is genital pain that occurs with intercourse.
• Vaginismus is an involuntary muscle spasm affecting the lower third of the vagina that occurs in response to any type of vaginal penetration of a sexual or nonsexual nature. These vaginal muscle spasms interfere with intercourse and can be painful.
• Noncoital sexual pain disorder is genital pain that occurs with any type of noncoital sexual stimulation.

Should you talk to your doctor if you are having sexual problems?

Interestingly, a lack of time is one of the most common reasons why health-care providers do not ask women about the possible presence of FSD. Women and their partners should feel comfortable discussing sexual health with their doctors. If their doctors do not routinely ask questions related to sexual health, women should inform their doctors if they are sexually active, having any problems with sexual activity, and/or having pain with intercourse.

Use of a Questionnaire

Women ought to be encouraged to discuss sexual problems and dysfunctions with their partners and doctors. When women suspect they may have FSD, it is a good idea for them to fill out a well-researched and validated online questionnaire such as the Female Sexual Function Index (FSFI). They can review the results with their doctor. The FSFI can be found on the Internet at www.fsfi-questionnaire.com. A total score of 26 or less on the FSFI indicates that the test taker may have FSD. The FSFI and other female sexual health questionnaires that cover information relevant to FSD, including the subtypes, are available at various locations online and offline. When individuals fill out questionnaires, their doctors are better able to detect, evaluate, and discuss with them information that may be critical to solving the problem.

Medical History

In order to determine if you may have FSD, it is very important for your doctor to perform a thorough medical history check. Some of the following conditions can affect sexual function:

- Hormonal issues, such as a reduction in estrogen or testosterone
- Cardiovascular disease and risk factors, including high cholesterol, high blood pressure, a lack of exercise, obesity, etc.
- Childbirth and pregnancy issues, such as a difficult vaginal delivery
- Contraceptives
- Diabetes
- Over-the-counter and prescription medications
- Alcohol and/or drug use
- Depression and other mental health issues
- Neurological issues
- Sleep issues
- Surgeries
- Tobacco use
- Thyroid disease
- Weight or waist gain

Physical and Mental Health Matter

Increased blood flow in the pelvic area and breasts and increased muscle tension in the body characterize the normal physical sexual response in females. When blood flow to the vagina increases, there is an increase in the vaginal secretions that are necessary to adequately lubricate the vagina for intercourse. Since the hormone estrogen helps with this response, low estrogen levels can result in a dramatic reduction in blood flow to the clitoris, vagina, and urethra, and this can cause these areas to thin. Any medication or medical condition that causes a problem in these areas can cause FSD. The treatment of physical issues that sometimes result in reduced sexual health, such as pain, incontinence, and low hormone levels, may improve sexual functioning. Stress, anxiety, depression, emotions, and past and present relationships and experiences all have important influences on the sexual process. Due to the importance of psychological well-being sexually and generally, mental health evaluation and discussion are critical.

Blood Tests

When looking for an explanation for sexual problems, it is not unusual for sexual health experts to test for hormone and other imbalances. Measuring the levels of hormones such as prolactin, thyroid, adrenal (DHEAS), estrogen, and testosterone may provide insight into sexual health. With or without estrogen, progesterone does not seem to have much of an impact on female sexual functioning. It may also be useful to measure markers of cardiovascular health such as cholesterol, hs-CRP, and glucose when looking at sexual issues.

Don't forget that every laboratory test comes with a catch! Just because the results of a blood test show nutrient or hormone levels to be high or low, this doesn't necessarily indicate the cause of a problem. Fall does not happen because summer ends. Just as the explanation of seasonal changes is far more complicated than summer simply fading into fall, your body is complex!

A health-care practitioner who carefully listens and combines information gathered from the questions, questionnaires, medical history, physical examination, mental health evaluation, and the results of all other tests is more likely to resolve an issue you may have than someone who diagnoses a problem based only on nutrient or hormone levels from blood tests. Unfortunately, blood test results are used to make diagnoses and treatment recommendations all the time in medicine without performing a more comprehensive assessment.

What treatments are available to treat FSD?

In my lifetime, virtually every drug that researchers thought would improve female sexual function has been rejected. Is there not enough money going to FSD research? Maybe. Is the treatment of female sexual issues more complex than it is with men? Maybe. Libido, arousal, and orgasm issues are common among women and are not easy to solve.

Lifestyle changes may help improve arousal in some women and could probably help with some other areas of FSD. Just increasing blood flow to a woman's genitals with a drug usually doesn't improve desire, arousal, or orgasm; the female sexual response involves neurovascular, hormonal, and psychological factors. Unless physical, mental, and emotional aspects of health are addressed, it is difficult to solve many desire, arousal, and orgasm issues.

FSD TREATMENTS

Bupropion

Bupropion is a dopamine receptor agonist, somewhat like Apomorphine, that is used to treat depression and improve mental health. This prescription drug is also used to help some people quit smoking! Some studies suggest it improves sexual desire and activity in women already negatively impacted sexually by antidepressant medication and perhaps even in some women who are not depressed. Bupropion has not received a glowing endorsement from some experts because the results have not been consistent. Some premenopausal women with hypoactive sexual desire disorder may experience increased arousal, orgasm completion, and sexual satisfaction using this medication.

Interestingly, Bupropion is being tested with another drug, Naltrexone, as a potential prescription weight-loss drug. Even though the majority of an advisory panel to the FDA voted in favor of approving it for weight reduction, it is not currently FDA approved as a weight-loss medication.

DHEA

DHEA is a dietary supplement that has controversial results when used at 25 mg to 50 mg. When using this supplement, pre- and postmenopausal women with hormonal deficiencies experienced an improvement in desire, arousal, orgasm, and sexual satisfaction. Recent larger studies have not been able to show DHEA to have benefits similar to those found in older studies. DHEA usually converts to testosterone or other androgens in postmenopausal women. Before you decide whether or not to take DHEA, please read the section below on testosterone and discuss this supplement with your doctor.

Estrogen

Estrogen and associated hormonal intravaginal creams, tablets, injections, and rings can increase vaginal lubrication by improving vaginal and clitoral blood flow, especially in postmenopausal women with genital pain and dryness issues. Menopause can cause the vaginal and vulvar tissue to become thin and easily irritated. Vaginal dryness, vaginitis, reduced labial sensation, and a reduction in desire all can occur when estrogen declines during menopause. These sexual problems can respond well to estrogen replacement. However, estrogen comes with an increased risk of certain cardiovascular diseases, especially when taken by older women and in pill form. Progesterone may need to be used to reduce the risk of endometrial cancer, but progesterone increases the risk of other medical conditions. You should discuss the use of hormone replacement therapy with your doctor because weighing the risks and benefits is an important consideration.

L-Arginine and L-Citrulline

A few previous studies of a combination supplement with L-arginine, ginseng, and other ingredients showed that it helped to improve arousal, desire, orgasm, sexual frequency, clitoral sensation, and increased sexual function scores. These findings mean that L-arginine and/or L-citrulline dietary supplementation may help in similar ways.

Lubricants

For the right candidate, lubricants that are water or glycerin based and those with L-arginine or L-citrulline may improve blood flow, desire, arousal, orgasm and pleasure. Talk to your doctor to see if using certain lubricants before sex may be helpful, or just give them a try and tell your doctor what happened.

Prostaglandin

Prostaglandin cream with alprostadil (the same drug used for penile pellet or injection therapy) contains the synthetic form of the natural prostaglandin E1 compound made by the human body. In studies, this drug is applied as a gel, cream, or liquid to the vulva and clitoris in order to increase blood flow to these areas and to increase vaginal lubrication and sexual arousal. This is not an FDA-approved drug, but you can still ask your doctor about the latest research if you are interested.

Testosterone

Testosterone treatment is very controversial and comes with serious potential side effects. Women who take testosterone treatment may experience abnormal cholesterol changes, liver problems, a potential increased risk of breast cancer (according to some), and masculine side effects that include acne, clitoral enlargement, hair growth on the body, a deeper voice, male pattern baldness, and the lack of an ability to admit when they are wrong and to ask for directions (just kidding on the last two).

If a doctor is trying simply to raise testosterone in a woman to the normal levels for her age, these side effects are rare. Only a small amount of testosterone is needed in women (about 10 percent of what men need or less). It is when testosterone is given in excess that women may experience bad consequences. Testosterone and other androgens are normally produced in women in small amounts in the adrenal glands, which sit on top of the kidneys, and the ovaries. DHEA, DHEAS, androstenedione and dihydrotestosterone (DHT) are other androgens produced by women that may affect sexual health.

There are plenty of companies willing to sell some of these compounds, so be careful. Women who get too much of these compounds, including testosterone, could change enough to have the w and o removed from the word woman, if you know what I mean!

Regardless, testosterone continues to be researched as a potential method of improving sexual desire and other areas of FSD, especially in women with very low levels of testosterone. Some interesting research shows that combining testosterone with estrogen may have some benefit for women who have experienced menopause due to the surgical removal of their ovaries.

Using testosterone to improve desire in women is very controversial and should be discussed with an expert. In my opinion, it is healthier to first lose weight if excess weight is an issue and see what happens before considering other options. In addition, emotional issues, relationship distress, life stress, and painful intercourse (dyspareunia) are all associated with low sexual desire in some women. Perhaps these potential contributors to low sexual desire should be dealt with first and foremost before considering more controversial treatments. Some experts even think that testosterone should not be prescribed until it is proven that testosterone does not cause breast cancer. Be very careful when weighing the risks and benefits of taking testosterone to improve desire.

Tibolone
This is a steroid approved in Europe that has estrogen, progesterone, and testosterone-like properties that may help some women with FSD. However, if you want this drug, you'll have to travel to Europe or locate a supplier.

Viagra
Viagra and other ED drugs increase genital blood flow and lubrication in women, but have not consistently helped women with FSD or worked better than a placebo. Maybe in the future there will be some women who see a benefit to using these drugs for sexual dysfunction from diabetes, arousal issues, an inability to get adequate genital blood flow, or issues related to prescription antidepressant use.

My last piece of advice for women will surprise you. It turns out that the heart-healthy tips we gave to men in Chapter Two work for FSD, too. Even though men and women are different in some ways, we are similar in others. As homework, I'd like women and men to turn back and reread Chapter two. Simple tips, such as exercising and diet changes, can make a big difference in your overall health as well as your sexual health. Don't forget Dr. Moyad's favorite mantra...

Heart Health = Sexual Health!

A final thought: when it comes to sexuality, don't be afraid to experiment a bit to see what gives you and your partner the most satisfaction. Whether it is a new supplement or medication, a new and interesting technique, or simply a new mindset, I hope that you realize as you read this book that there are many, many options available to give you a healthier, happier sex life. Enjoy!

Appendix

Dr. Moyad's Tips for Improving Sexual Function and Boosting Nitric Oxide (NO)

Following are a collection of tips aimed at improving any man's or woman's chance of maintaining or improving his or her sexual function. Even men who have had some form of prostate surgery or women who have had a medical procedure that may affect their sexual health may also benefit from these tips. Most of the tips have one common element: they help in some way to increase blood levels of nitric oxide (NO), one of the primary compounds produced by the body that improves sexual health. You may find that trying even one or two of the tips will help improve your sexual interest, function, and overall satisfaction.

TIP 1
Take the time to fill out a medically oriented sexual health questionnaire.

Find a validated questionnaire. They are generally available for download on the Internet or at physicians' offices. Fill one out and review your results with your doctor. Many sexual health experts encourage men to fill out the International Index of Erectile Function (IIEF) questionnaire. It is my favorite because it also covers libido as well, and it includes 15 questions. Two others, the Sexual Health Inventory for Men (SHIM, 5 questions) or Erection Hardness Score (EHS, 1 question), can also be used. Men who have had prostate surgery may also want to talk to their doctors about completing an Expanded Prostate Cancer Index Composite (EPIC) questionnaire.

Women should fill out the Female Sexual Function Index (FSFI) or another one recommended by their doctor. These questionnaires can help determine the changes over time in your sexual health (sort of like a cholesterol test for sexual health).

duce your cardiovascular risk to as close to zero as possible.

A few things to consider in reducing your risk:
- Do not allow any part of your cholesterol or cardiovascular disease blood tests to be abnormal (LDL, HDL, triglycerides or hs-CRP).
- Maintain a normal blood pressure,
- Maintain a normal blood glucose level.
- No tobacco products (that includes cigars and chewing tobacco).
- Exercise at least every other day for 30 minutes or more (break a sweat).
- Lift upper and lower body weights 2 to 3 times a week.
- Lose some weight and/or waist.
- Follow a Mediterranean Diet plan or another plant-based heart-healthy diet.
- Stay away from any type of alcohol in excess

TIP 3
Make your mental health as much of a priority as your physical health.

Anything that negatively affects your mental health should be addressed through lifestyle changes, supplements, medications, therapy, etc. It is a fact that depression can be improved by exposure to light, socializing, exercise, some supplements (SAM-e, fish oil, flaxseed, etc.), numerous prescription drugs, and counseling or therapy. Stress and anxiety should be reduced by exercises, some supplements (such as L-theanine), prescription medications, and counseling or therapy. Sleeping 7 to 8 hours a night can improve your mental state, too. It is a little-known fact that lack of sleep reduces sexual hormones (not to mention interest in sex, I suspect).

TIP 4
Do not be afraid to take a pill(s) or use other medical interventions to improve your sexual health.

Ego aside, there are a number of options that truly help individuals. From prescription ED medications to supplements to devices or injections—there are many to consider to find one that works best for you. I will offer a word of caution to use care that the devices particularly are medically approved (including safety features) and that the supplements are tested to be pure and safe. As we have noted, lots of supplement products contain unsafe or contaminated ingredients. Some on the market, such as Triverex, offer quality tested ingredients and are safe to use, while others may contain unsafe combinations of compounds.

Worth noting here are non-medical items that may enhance sexual experiences, such as sexual toys and lubricants. While not exactly in the same category as medical interventions, they can, if chosen carefully, make for more enjoyable sexual experiences. At times, something as simple as a personal lubricant can resolve an issue.

TIP 5
Do not be afraid to speak with your doctor about removing or reducing a pill or pills to improve sexual health.

Over-the-counter pain medications, some supplements, and many prescription pills can reduce sexual function. Review your over-the-counter and prescription list with your doctor to see if any of them can be reduced or eliminated.

TIP 6
Talk to a trusted health-care professional or specialist (a urologist or sex therapist, for example) for the latest advice and therapies.

An expert on sexual health can review blood flow, hormonal changes, nerve function, and even mental health. Because so many things affect sexual health, a proper evaluation and individual history is a start to finding help. Life is too short not to see a sexual health specialist if you are having physical and/or mental health problems that are affecting your sexual health. Now, more than ever, help is out there!